Let's stay in touch.

Please send us this card so that we can keep you informed.

☐ Please send me 10 issues of *Smart Drug News*, the newsletter of cognition enhancement; a free product sources list; and your directory of physicians. Enclosed is $44 ($46 Canada/Mexico, $55 overseas).

☐ Please send me a product sources list and your directory of physicians. Enclosed is $2 and a self-addressed stamped envelope.

☐ I am a physician. Please add me to your directory. (*Physicians: please describe your practice.*)

☎ Phone orders call 415-321-CERI, FAX 415-323-3864.

Name _____

Company _____

Address _____

City _____ State _____ Zip _____

Credit   Exp.
card # _____ date _____

Visa / MC

Signature _____

Answer these questions only if you want to.
Are you a health professional? ☐ Yes ☐ No
What is your age? ☐ under 30 ☐ 30-50 ☐ 50+
Yearly income? ☐ under $40K ☐ $40-100K ☐ $100K+

Please let us know about your experiences with smart drugs and nutrients (use a separate sheet if necessary).

_____

_____

_____

_____

D0189336

_____

ERi P. O. Box 4029–2014
Menlo Park, CA 94026–4029

Cognitive Enhancement Research Institute

P.O. Box 4029–2014

Menlo Park, CA 94026–4029

Let's stay in touch.

Please mail us this page so that we can keep you informed.

☐ Please send me 10 issues of *Smart Drug News*, the newsletter of cognition enhancement; a free product sources list; and your directory of physicians. Enclosed is $44 ($46 Canada/Mexico, $55 overseas).

☐ Please send me a product sources list and your directory of physicians. Enclosed is $2 and a self-addressed stamped envelope.

☐ I am a physician. Please add me to your directory. (*Physicians: please describe your practice.*)

☎ Phone orders call 415-321-CERI, FAX: 415-323-3864.

Name _____

Company _____

Address _____

City _____ State _____ Zip _____

Credit
card # _____ Exp.
date _____

Visa / MC

Signature _____

Answer these questions only if you want to.
Are you a health professional? ☐ Yes ☐ No
What is your age? ☐ under 30 ☐ 30-50 ☐ 50+
Yearly income? ☐ under $40K ☐ $40-100K ☐ $100K+

Please let us know about your experiences with smart drugs and nutrients (use a separate sheet if necessary).

_____

_____

_____

_____

Mail this page to:
CERI, P.O. Box 4029-2014, Menlo Park, CA 94026-4029.

What Others are Saying About *Smart Drugs & Nutrients* and *Smart Drugs II*

"...a fascinating and controversial subject..."
> Barbara Walters, ABC *Nightline*

"...a bible for the smart drug set."
> *Los Angeles Times Magazine*

"...an excellent introduction to the field of cognition-enhancing compounds... well-written and easily understood, even by people who do not have specific training in medicine."
> Giacomo Spignoli, M.D., Ph.D.
> Pharmacology Research Director
> L. Manetti-H. Roberts & Co.

"...opens up the new world of nootropics..."
> Ernest Lawrence Rossi, Ph.D.
> Author of *The Psychobiology of Mind-Body Healing*

"...a very important book. Very interesting and well documented...an absolutely essential and important subject."
> Timothy Leary, Ph.D.

"...an easy book to read and very interesting. I recommend it to any consumer who wants to be better informed and take more control over his or her own health."
> Cliff Wong, R.Ph.

"...a dirty little book."
> Dan Rowland, Compliance Officer
> Los Angeles District Office
> Food and Drug Administration

"...a wonderful self-help manual... I was especially pleased with the section regarding smart drugs and the law. Physicians wanting to prescribe these drugs will find this section very useful."
> Robert Buckley, M.D.

Other Books by the Authors

Smart Drugs & Nutrients
by Ward Dean, M.D., and John Morgenthaler
Volume 1 in the Smart Drug Series (Health Freedom Publications, 1990).

STOP the FDA: Save Your Health Freedom
edited by John Morgenthaler and Steven Wm. Fowkes
An expose of the FDA's campaign against health freedom in America (Health Freedom Publications, 1992).

The Neuroendocrine Theory of Aging
and Degenerative Disease
by Vladimir M. Dilman, M.D., Ph.D., D. M. Sc.,
and Ward Dean, M.D.
An explanation of the neuroendocrine mechanisms of aging and their relationship to developmental and degenerative processes. Intended for medical professionals and sophisticated lay readers. Edited and illustrated by Steven Wm. Fowkes (Center for Bio-Gerontology, 1991).

Biological Aging Measurement — Clinical Applications
by Ward Dean
A worldwide survey of aging-measurement systems with detailed discussion of the age-related physiological parameters which serve as biomarkers. (Center for Bio-Gerontology, 1988).

Commonly Asked Questions About Smart Drugs and Nutrients

During 1991 and 1992, we gave about 300 interviews with journalists and spoke with hundreds of other people about our book, *Smart Drugs & Nutrients*. We noticed that almost everyone asked the same basic questions. For your convenience, we list them here with some very quick answers (see our Q&A section for in-depth answers to many questions).

Q. What are smart drugs and nutrients?

These are substances that enhance physical or mental performance with few unwanted side effects. Some are pharmaceuticals and some are natural nutrients or herbs.

Q. What effects do people notice from taking smart drugs?

People can experience improvements in memory, IQ, reaction time, mood, energy level, sensory perception, sexual arousal and response, music appreciation, and more. The intensity of effect varies greatly from person to person and drug to drug, and can range from no perceptible effect at all to a profound life-transformation. Most people get a noticeable enough effect that they choose to continue using smart drugs. (See the chapter called "Smart Drug Users" for first-hand accounts).

Q. Are smart drugs safe?

Anything can be unsafe if misused. However, research indicates that smart drugs are among the safest drugs in the world, and are quite safe when compared to commonly used substances such as coffee and aspirin. Many smart drugs have other health benefits, and some may even extend lifespan.

Q. What happens when you stop taking smart drugs? Do you get dumb?

No dumber than when you started. Most effects subside after a few weeks, leaving you back where you started, but no worse.

Q. **What smart drugs & nutrients do you take? How long have you been taking smart drugs?**

We've all been using various smart drugs and nutrients for different situations for more than a decade.

Q. **Are smart drugs addictive?**

No.

Q. **How do you know that smart drugs work?**

We know smart drugs work for a number of reasons. First, because published scientific studies (many of which we cite in this book) prove it. There have been thousands of such studies conducted all over the world for the past 40 years. Second, we have had countless positive anecdotal reports from our readers, friends, and patients. Third, we have experienced the results ourselves.

Q. **Do any studies show that smart drugs work on normal, healthy humans?**

Many. We focus on them in this book. The reason that there are not more studies with normal people is that drugs are usually designed to cure illnesses, and are therefore tested on sick people.

Q. **Do smart drugs work for senility or Alzheimer's disease?**

Yes, if they are administered early in the course of the disease. In the following chapters, we describe many studies which confirm the effectiveness of smart drugs for these conditions. (See the chapter called "Suggested Treatment Protocol for Alzheimer's Disease".)

Q. **How do smart drugs compare with anabolic steroids?**

Like anabolic steroids, smart drugs are *performance enhancers*. Unlike steroids, they have few or no known negative side effects.

Q. **How do smart drugs compare with recreational drugs?**

There is little comparison. Smart drugs enhance performance, without causing euphoria or dysfunction. Smart drugs are also non-addictive, and may even improve your health.

Q. **How many people would you say are using smart drugs?**

ABC's *Nightline* estimated there were over 100,000 users in the U.S. in 1991. We now estimate that there are over a million smart drug users worldwide, based on sales figures from pharmaceutical companies.

Q. **Is there a smart drug sub-culture developing?**

Yes, but it is not "the 60s revisited." Smart drug people are pragmatic, performance-oriented individuals of every age and demographic group seeking personal enhancement through high technology and hard science. Young smart drug advocates may take them to get better grades. Baby-boomers may take them to maintain a competitive edge in their business or professional lives. Older smart drug users may take them to ward off age-associated memory impairment (AAMI). Those with actual cognition-impairing conditions like Alzheimer's disease or Parkinson's disease, of course, take various smart drugs for treatment, often on the advice of their physicians.

Smart Drugs II
The Next Generation

**New Drugs and Nutrients
to Improve Your Memory and
Increase Your Intelligence**

By
Ward Dean, M.D.,
John Morgenthaler, and
Steven Wm. Fowkes

Health Freedom Publications
P.O. Box 2515
Menlo Park, CA 94026

Volume 2 in the Smart Drug Series

Smart Drugs II: The Next Generation

New Drugs and Nutrients to Improve Your Memory and
Increase Your Intelligence

By Ward Dean, M.D.,
John Morgenthaler, and
Steven Wm. Fowkes

Published by
Health Freedom Publications
P.O. Box 2515 — Menlo Park, CA 94026

Library of Congress Catalog Card Number: 93-78074
First Printing 1993
Printed in the United States of America
First Edition

Library of Congress Cataloging in Publication Data
Dean, Ward.
Smart Drugs II: The Next Generation — New Drugs and
Nutrients to Improve Your Memory and Increase Your
Intelligence / by Ward Dean, M.D., John Morgenthaler, and
Steven Wm. Fowkes.
　　Includes references and index.
　　1. Intellect—nutritional aspects.
　　2. Neuropharmacology.
　　3. Brain—aging prevention.
　　4. Health.
　　5. Memory.
　　6. Alzheimer's disease.
QP398.D44　　1993　　153.9-dc20　　CIP 93-78074
ISBN: 0-9627418-7-6:　$14.95 Softcover

Table of Contents

Acknowledgements

Special thanks go to the following individuals: William Keith Powell for his crucial role in creating and editing this book; T. Michael Hardy, Assistant Editor for *Smart Drug News*; and Associate Editor Sunah Cherwin.

We would also like to thank: Steve All; Chris Andreae; Henry Andreae; Ian Andreae; Max Andreae; Dave Aujus; Willem J. Baars; Freddy Baer & the Baer clan; Walter Baron; Michelle Barnett; Deborah Benner; Alison Benney; Arne Bey; Sally Binford, Ph.D.; Will Block; Deborah Bourienne; Bridget Byrd; Bob Buckley, M.D.; Rue Burlingham; Tammy Burwell; Dede Callichy; Jeffrey Devon Card; Hyla Cass, M.D.; Ewai Chan; Amy Coffman; Henry Dakin; Steve Davis; Kris Dean; Kumja Dean; Nancy Denenberg; Beverly DesChaux; Troy Dickerson; Magi Discoe; Ryan Donovan; Karla Downing; Jack Dreyfus; the EgoSoft gang (Grandee Arthur Fermont, Rodica Harabagiu, *et al.*); Cassandra English; Jim English; Claire Farr; Laura Fast; Nancy Frank; John Furber; Ken Goffman; Ira Goldberg; Flash Gordon, M.D.; Hilary Hamm; Ann Harry; Kevin Hull; Michael Hutchison; Mike Hyson, Ph.D.; InfoSelect; John S. James; Richard Kaufman, Ph.D.; Alison Kennedy; Dharma Singh Khalsa, M.D.; Ron Klatz, D.O.; Gerald Larson; Sherry Lynesther; Jeff Mandel; Robert McDonald; Romany McNamara; Maggi MacLean; Clinton Ray & Bonnie K. Miller; Samantha Miller; Michael Mooney; Pat, Fred, and Wayne Morgenthaler; Burl T. Moss; Ethel Neal; Tom Nufert; Sebastian Orfali; Scott Paddor; Babs Patton; Durk Pearson; Ross Pelton, R.Ph., Ph.D.; Taffy Clarke Pelton; Judy Pincus; Curtis Ponzi; Beverly Potter; Betty Powell; Dan Poynter; Mike Pratter and Pratter, Gardner, & Graves; William Regelson, M.D.; Mark Rennie; Kathryn Roberts; Larry Roberts; Michael Rosenbaum, M.D.; R. Rucker; Luc Sala; Sandoz Pharmaceuticals; Curtis Schreier; Sandy Shaw; Helen Silver; George Sisson; Jeremy Slate; Diana Smith; Maurice W. H. L. M. Snellen; James South; Giacomo Spignoli, M.D.; Arnold Stillman; Barry Stinson; Robert THK Trossel, M.D.; UCB Pharmaceuticals; Lorna Vanderhaeghe; Jim Warshauer; Day Waterbury; Julie Weber; M. E. "Killa" White-Pillow; Cricket Wingfield, M.D.; and Gordon Withrow.

Disclaimer

This book is not intended to provide medical advice. It is intended to be used for educational and informational purposes only.

Although most of the substances discussed in this book are remarkably free from adverse side effects, combinations of these substances alone or with other nutrients or drugs may have unknown adverse effects. We recommend consulting with a knowledgeable physician before embarking on a cognition enhancement program.

Introduction

Prior to the publication of *Smart Drugs & Nutrients* in 1991, no references to the term "smart drug" could be found in a computer search of thirty of the largest newspapers in America. Although several excellent books had focused, more or less, on the use of drugs and nutrients for performance enhancement, the term "smart drugs" had not entered the popular lexicon.

Smart Drugs & Nutrients, however, fired the imaginations of journalists. In one year, the authors were featured on the *Today* show, CNN's *Larry King Live*, *20/20*, *Donahue*, Australian *60 Minutes*, and many other major television and radio talk shows. Hundreds of newspaper articles appeared in Europe, Asia, Latin America, Canada, England and Australia. Many prestigious American newspapers and magazines featured stories about smart drugs. For example, the *San Francisco Chronicle* had eleven articles alone, and the *Washington Post* carried seven. *Smart Drugs & Nutrients* was also featured in articles in *Time*, *Playboy*, *USA Today*, the *Washington Post*, the *New York Times*, the *Los Angeles Times*, *The Economist*, *Worth*, *Rolling Stone*, *Mademoiselle*, and many other publications.

Smart Drugs & Nutrients sold a respectable 70,000 copies in its first two years. For a highly technical, non-fiction reference book, this is considered a mega-success in the publishing world.

What are Smart Drugs, Anyway?

What exactly is a smart drug? The most common meaning that comes to mind for the word "smart" is "intelligent." Smart people are mentally alert and bright, or witty and clever. But what *exactly* are we talking about with such descriptive phrases? Are we talking about intelligence and abstract reasoning? Are we also including memory? How about cognition? Coordination and dexterity? Sensory perception? Musical talent? Reaction time? Or what about something really esoteric, like the ability to appreciate a joke or pun, or a sense of life as a wonderful adventure?

All of these aspects of mental function are important to us in different ways and to different degrees. Rather than deal with smart drugs only within the narrow contexts of cognition, intelligence, and memory, we will deal with all aspects of mental performance. Within this expanded context, any drug or nutrient which enhances aspects of mental performance can be considered a "smart" drug or nutrient.

When we speak of "cognitive enhancement," we wish to include all the myriad mental functions that go into making us what we are. This would not only include such obvious functions as intelligence and memory, but those such as sex, relaxation, sleep, immune function, and neuroendocrine regulation. These are all vital aspects of human health and well-being which are intimately related to the functioning of the brain.

A Change in World View

In 1992, *Time* magazine published a feature article about vitamins. The cover boldly proclaimed, "New evidence shows they may help fight cancer, heart disease, and the ravages of aging." Ten years ago, such a statement would not have been made by a mainstream publication. Although this comment would have been just as true then, few scientists took nutrient supplements seriously, much less *internally*. At a recent gerontological conference, one attendee commented that nearly everyone in the field is now using at least some supplements. Americans spend $3.3 billion on vitamins and nutrients every year — and that figure is growing. When comedian Martin Short complained, "I can't remember" on the television show *Late Night With David Letterman*, Dave snorted, "You're not getting enough lecithin!" Taking supplements is now mainstream, and only a few fringe types unfamiliar with the research still think that they are worthless.

We are now at a similar place with smart drugs as we were 10 years ago with vitamins. That is, we're a few years away from total public acceptance and 20 years away from bureaucratic acceptance. Smart drugs are becoming part of our consensus reality.

The Media Shift Gears

Until early 1993, the smart drug media spectacle focused on the question: do smart drugs work or are they just snake oil? This is the point around which all journalists seemingly attempted to remain 'balanced.' But it is only the first in a series of pivotal issues which will ultimately change the way we think about drugs and cognitive enhancement. The "do they work?" question has been answered. Today's questions are: should individuals enhance their mental performance? What are the social benefits and consequences of smart-drug use? Is smart-drug use fair? Is it ethical?

Dr. James M. Ellison, director of psychopharmacology at New England Medical Center in Boston, noted in *Family Practice News* and in *Psychiatric Times* that it *is* considered ethical to perform cosmetic plastic surgery, treat normal hair loss, and prevent injuries and improve performance through sports medicine. According to Dr. Ellison, these types of "medical health enhancement" are ethically similar to the use of smart drugs.

To Enhance or Not to Enhance?

Are smart-drug critics objecting the use of smart drugs or are they really objecting to personal enhancement? Many of us wish to enhance ourselves as individuals, but is it okay for others to do the same? Will smart-drug use be socially acceptable?

We agree with Dr. Ellison that enhancing ourselves with smart drugs and nutrients is similar to enhancing ourselves with better diets, vitamin regimens, exercise programs, employment experiences, and ongoing educational courses. Giving vitamins

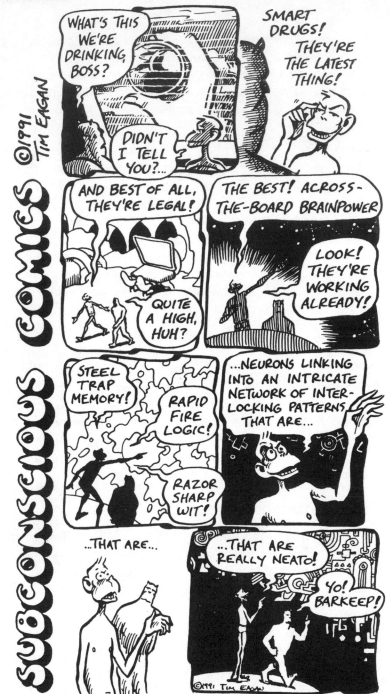

to children to increase their non-verbal intelligence (see the Vitamin Update chapter) is exactly analogous to pregnant women taking prenatal vitamins to deliver healthier babies. The ethics of such situations are quite clear to us; it is the choice of each individual to decide his or her path to better health, wisdom and enlightenment.

Many smart-drug critics decry the dangers of smart drugs. We could repeat our discussions about the relative safety of smart drugs (*i.e.*, smart drugs are safer than aspirin), but the real question is: should people be allowed to endanger themselves (at all) for the sake of enhancement? We think so. Most people don't think twice about the risks of driving to the grocery store, crossing the street, or taking a Tylenol for a headache. Will we create restrictive social policy about risks of this magnitude? We hope not.

Smart Drugs to Become Big Business in the 90s

According to *The Economist*, the weekly newsmagazine from England, "the American pharmaceutical industry is developing more than 140 types of smart pills in its laboratories, making them the tenth-largest class of drugs being researched." Ciba-Geigy, one of Japan's largest pharmaceutical companies, projects $50 million in annual sales for just one drug, oxiracetam. *Fortune* magazine speculated that total smart drug sales could top $1 billion per year within a few years. In fact, in 1990 the pharmaceutical giant UCB reported $1 billion in world-wide sales for piracetam (see the Piracetam Update chapter). *Worth* magazine quoted David Saks, a senior drug analyst for Wedbush Morgan Securities: "You can see the possibility of 10, 20, 50 million healthy Americans using drugs to enhance memory functions, and that's a very large investment opportunity."

Drug companies do their work by targeting a particular disease and then developing a drug which will deal with that disease. This is because the legal procedure for drug development is disease-oriented. There is no current legal basis for approving drugs for performance enhancement. Performance-enhancing drugs can be approved, but only if they can be demonstrated effective for the treatment of some disease. Drug companies can, however, define a new disease or redefine an old disease.

These days, drug companies want to broaden their market by defining a new disease called 'age-associated memory impairment' (AAMI) [Amaducci, *et al.*, 1992; Crook, *et al.*, 1986; Crook, 1992; Leber, 1992; Raffaele, *et al.*, 1992]. Once AAMI is defined as a disease, it will become a legitimate target for drug development and, eventually, approval. Nearly every drug company is in the race to develop drugs for AAMI.

According to Dr. James McGaugh of the Center for Neurobiology of Learning and Memory:

"It doesn't take a smart pill to...realize that there is a large market for people who want to have their memories improved. Certainly, there is a large market with Alzheimer's disease alone. There is an even larger market if you consider people who have other forms of memory disorder. And then, there is an absolutely huge market for people who believe that their lives would be better if they could only remember a little bit better. Now who's going to be the one to tell them that they can't take this pill?"

Dr. Paul Williams, Director of CNS Clinical Research at Glaxo Pharmaceuticals, explains the concept.

"I guess we can all think of eighty-year-olds whose memories are crystal clear. On the other hand, there are people in their early 50s who have difficulty remembering telephone numbers, maybe difficulty in remembering names, difficulty putting names to faces. For some of these people their memory impairment interferes with their functioning — interferes with the way they carry out their jobs, maybe interferes with aspects of their social life. And it is when we have memory impairment to that degree that we speak of age-associated memory impairment."

According to Professor Ian Hindmarch of the University of Surrey's Human Psychopharmacology Research Unit, more than 160 cognition-enhancement drugs are in development worldwide. The top category of drug development, anti-cancer agents, comprises only about 260 drugs worldwide.

Professor Hindmarch predicts that, "...if they could invent a disorder that could be improved by a cognitive enhancer, then, in fact, this is bonanza time, this is printing money!"

"There will be more than one billion-dollar drug that comes into this market in the next decade," says Stover Haley Noyes analyst Rick Stover. "And all the major companies want to own them."

When asked why Glaxo is developing drugs for AAMI rather than Alzheimer's Disease, Paul Williams answered with a definite gleam in his eye:

> *Age-associated memory impairment affects very many more people than Alzheimer's disease, although, it's certainly true, it is a much less severe condition. We believe that at least 4 million people in the U.K. suffer from age-associated memory impairment. So if [a treatment] is eventually made available to them, there will be an awful lot of people very interested indeed.*

How Much Research is Really Going On?

We wanted to have a picture that would represent the increase of interest in smart drugs over the past 20 years, so we developed some statistics using Medline (the computer version of the National Library of Medicine) and Embase (the computer version of the European medical library). The graphs below plot the number of papers published each year which mentioned the smart drugs piracetam and deprenyl.

It is interesting to note that piracetam is not investigated for much of anything *except* cognition enhancement. There does not appear to be much chance of its approval in the U.S. for treatment of Alzheimer's disease. Also, since the patents on piracetam have expired, drug companies don't have much incentive to pump research money into it. Deprenyl's patent has also expired.

These graphs reflect the progressively increasing interest in smart drugs among the scientific research community.

Age-Associated Memory Impairment

In *Smart Drugs & Nutrients*, we wrote of age-related mental decline or ARMD. Now we have a new term: age-associated memory impairment or AAMI (see the graph at the top of page 26). Both terms are attempts to quantify the age-related loss of cognitive functioning. AAMI is more specific than ARMD, focusing solely on the memory-related aspects of this multi-

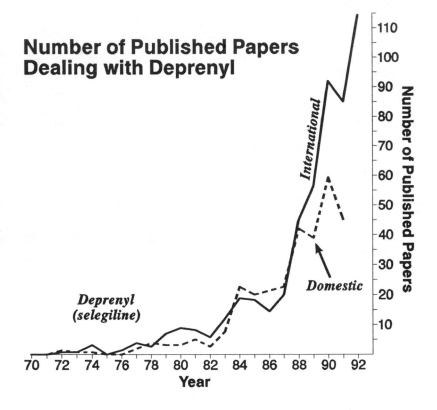

Number of Published Papers Dealing with Deprenyl

faceted phenomenon. This specificity makes AAMI easier to measure. It also makes it easier for drug companies to establish the efficacy of a smart drug in treating AAMI. We expect to be hearing a lot more about AAMI in the coming years.

The FDA, under current law, can only approve drugs for *disease conditions*. If aging is not a disease, then no drugs can be approved for its treatment. However, if AAMI is designated to be a diagnosable and treatable disease, we may well be on the way to cutting the bureaucratic red tape with which the FDA has attempted to place a stranglehold on smart drug research and access in this country. If AAMI is a disease, then maybe

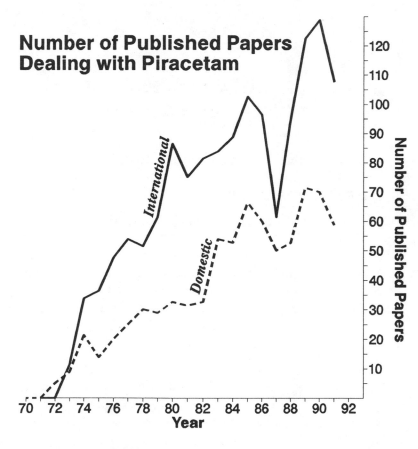

Number of Published Papers Dealing with Piracetam

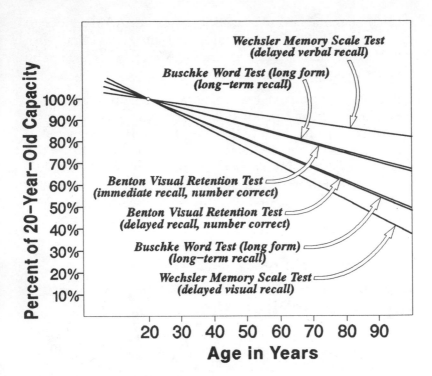

ARMD is a disease. And if ARMD is a disease, then maybe aging itself is a disease for which treatments could be approved.

The Next Generation

This book and its companion, *Smart Drugs & Nutrients*, are guides to this fascinating new science. In *Smart Drugs II*, we've included the latest discoveries about some of the drugs that were covered in *Smart Drugs & Nutrients* and new drugs which are now emerging into clinical practice throughout the world. *Smart Drugs II* has a full chapter of Questions & Answers — the most popular feature of our *Smart Drug News* newsletter. In that chapter are the questions asked by real smart drug users, and answers from our team.

We've also included a chapter about people who use smart drugs. We know that their stories don't constitute "proof" of anything, in the scientific sense of proof. Nevertheless, the stories are interesting, and researchers should read these stories with open minds. All scientific innovation begins with simple observation, and these are observations of people living on the cutting edge of science.

Smart Drugs II will inform you of the latest sources for smart drugs and nutrients, information, and professional medical assistance.

We've included fewer animal studies in this book than in our earlier book. This is because there are many more human studies now than when we did our research three years ago. When we do include animal studies, it's primarily to indicate where the research will go next.

How to Use Smart Drugs

Please read the following carefully. Every smart drug we've studied seems to have an inverted-U-shaped dose-response curve [Heiby, 1988]. This means that enough is enough, too little is too little, and too much may have an effect opposite of what you desire. We would like to be able to tell you the exact dosage needed for each smart substance. Unfortunately, we can't. The effects of smart substances are highly individualized. Only you, working with your physician, can determine the exact dosage that is right for you. And only you can determine which smart drugs and nutrients enhance your performance.

Start with only one new smart drug or nutrient at a time. Start with a low dose — substantially lower than what you think may be necessary. Pay attention to the effects. Does it work for you? Ask other people to observe your behavior and performance. Sometimes others see what we do not. The key point to keep in mind is that *everyone is different*. What works well for one person may not do anything for someone else. This is similar to the way various cold pills or anti-hypertensive medications may work for one person, but not another.

Asking selected friends, co-workers and family members to notice and comment on any changes in your behavior is an important option that many people do not fully utilize. We've seen one friend's verbal skills improve dramatically every time she tries piracetam, but she never notices the change until someone else comments on it. Another man didn't notice that the day after starting melatonin, he stopped taking his regular afternoon naps — until others asked him about it. These are only a couple of examples.

This book is *not* intended to provide medical advice. It is intended to be used for educational and informational purposes only. Although most of the substances discussed in this book are remarkably free from adverse side effects, combinations of these substances alone or with other nutrients or drugs may have unknown adverse effects. We recommend consulting with a knowledgeable physician before embarking on a cognition enhancement program of your own design. This is not a legal formality! Under no circumstances should this book be used as a substitute for medical advice.

References

Amaducci L, Lippi A, Bracco L and Falcini M. Definition and classification of age-related cognitive dysfunction. In: *Treatment of Age-Related Cognitive Dysfunction: Pharmacological and Clinical Evaluation*, by Racagni G and Mendlewicz J (Eds), Karger, Basel, 1992.

Bartus T, Dean RL, Sherman KA, Friedman E and Beer B. Profound effects of combining choline and piracetam on memory enhancement and cholinergic function in aged rats. *Neurobiology of Aging*. Vol. 2, pp. 105-11, 1981.

Bylinsky G. Medicine's Next Marvel: The Memory Pill. *Fortune*, pp. 68-72, 20 January 1986.

Crook TH, Bartus RT, Ferris SH, Whitehouse P, Cohen GD and Gershon S. Age-associated memory impairment: Proposed diagnostic criteria and measures of clinical change — report of a National Institute of Mental Health work group. *Dev Neuropsychol* 2: 261-76, 1986.

Crook TH. Assessment of clinical efficacy of cognitive enhancers. In: *Treatment of Age-Related Cognitive Dysfunction: Pharmacological and Clinical Evaluation*, by Racagni G and Mendlewicz J (Eds), Karger, Basel, 1992.

Debrovner D. Wising Up To Smart Drugs. *American Druggist*, pp. 34-43, December 1992

Economist, The. Don't Go Gaga, Be Like Babar. Pp. 81-2, 2 February 1991.

Ellison, James M. Cosmedication: A psychopharmacologic trend for the '90s. *Psychiatric Times* February 1993.

Fuller RB. *Synergetics*. New York: Macmillan Publishing, 1975.

Heiby WA. *The Reverse Effect*. Deerfield, Illinois: Mediscience Publishers, 1988.

Late Night With David Letterman, February 26, 1993.

Leber P. Developing pharmacological treatment for age-associated cognitive impairments: A regulatory perspective. In: *Treatment of Age-Related Cognitive Dysfunction: Pharmacological and Clinical Evaluation*, by Racagni G and Mendlewicz J (Eds), Karger, Basel, 1992.

Raffaele KC, Haxby JV and Schapiro MB. Age-Associated Memory Impairment. In: *Treatment of Age-Related Cognitive Dysfunction: Pharmacological and Clinical Evaluation*, by Racagni G and Mendlewicz J (Eds), Karger, Basel, 1992.

Schaffler K and Klausnitzer W. Randomized placebo-controlled double-blind crossover study on antihypoxidotic effects of piracetam using psychophysiological measures in healthy volunteers. *Arzneim Forsch* 38: 288-91, 1988.

Schoenthaler SJ, Moody JM and Pankow LD. Applied nutrition and behavior. *Journal of Applied Nutrition* 43(1): 31-9, 1991.

Tayman J. "Smart Drugs: The Next Big Thing?" *Worth*, pp. 90-95, August/September 1992.

Time magazine. Vitamins: New evidence shows they may help fight cancer, heart disease, and ravages of aging. April 6, 1992.

A Note for Beginners

If increasing your intelligence and enhancing your performance (and, just possibly, extending your lifespan) are novel concepts for you, welcome. Please read on and satisfy your curiosity. We hope you will act in deliberate and calculated ways as you step into your adventure.

Part I of this book includes a number of chapters reviewing different smart drugs and nutrients. These chapters are fairly technical and are intended as reference material. If you are new to the subject of smart drugs, we recommend that you first read the chapter called "Smart Drug Users" in Part II. This chapter will give you a much better feel for what smart drugs and smart drugs users are all about.

If you still have questions after reading this book, you can mail your questions to the Q&A Section of *Smart Drug News*. To subscribe, send in the tear-out card at the front of this book, or call 1-415-321-CERI.

Part I:

Smart Drugs
The Next Generation

Part I: Smart Drugs: The Next Generation

Deprenyl:
The Anti-Aging Smart Drug

Deprenyl (trade names Eldepryl, Jumex) was developed by Professor József Knoll of Semmelweis University in Hungary. It has been extensively researched since the 1950s and has been used by millions as a treatment for Parkinson's disease. Recently, deprenyl has been recognized as one of the most promising (and safe) drugs for treating Alzheimer's disease. Deprenyl is also one of the first drugs proven to extend maximum lifespan in animals, and it has been found to act as a cognition-enhancer in normal, healthy animals. As a bonus, deprenyl also acts as an aphrodisiac in male animals and some men. Because it corrects so many of the typical problems associated with aging we can justifiably call it an "anti-aging" drug.

Sex Enhancement

We have received a steady stream of reports from men (usually over age 50) who note increased libido after taking deprenyl. This is not surprising, considering the number of animal studies that have consistently shown dramatic increases in the sexual activity of old male rats (see the graph on page 37 [Knoll, *et al.*, 1983]). As far as we know, there have been no studies of deprenyl's aphrodisiac effects on normal, healthy humans, although our anecdotal reports would seem to indicate that human experimental results would parallel those of animal studies.

Life Extension Effects of Deprenyl

The oldest living humans live to about 110-120 years. This is the maximum lifespan for humans under normal conditions. However, the average human lives to be only about 70 or 80.

The maximum lifespan in rats is about 140 weeks (approximately three years), but the average life expectancy is, of course, considerably less than that. To extend the average lifespan means to increase the number of rats living to be older than the average. Many substances have been shown to extend

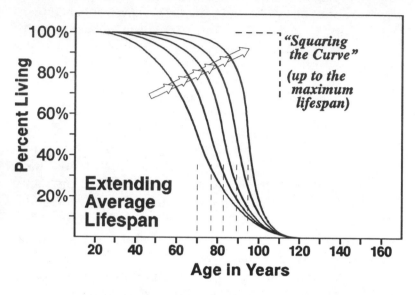

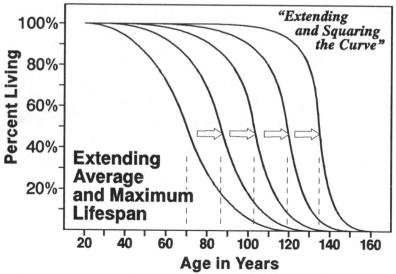

the average lifespan of laboratory animals (for example, vitamin E and BHT). Some scientists think these substances may also increase the odds of humans reaching closer to the maximum lifespan of 110-120 years.

Deprenyl, on the other hand, has been shown to extend maximum lifespan in rats by about 40%! This would be like a human living to 150 years of age! And if the animal research holds true for humans, a hundred-year-old would look and feel 60.

The graph above illustrates a normal survival curve and how that curve changes with life-extension techniques that increase average lifespans. As the average lifespan is increased, death is postponed to later ages and the survival curve (white arrows) becomes progressively "squarer," approaching the dashed-line maximum. With average-lifespan increases, the maximum lifespan is not increased, but a greater percentage of the population approaches the maximum age.

The bottom graph (facing page) illustrates the effect of a generalized slowing of the aging process itself, where both average *and* maximum lifespan are increased. Deprenyl has extended both average and maximum lifespan in animal studies.

The figure below depicts the dramatic lifespan increase in old rats treated with deprenyl, compared to placebo-treated controls. Note that all of the control animals had died well

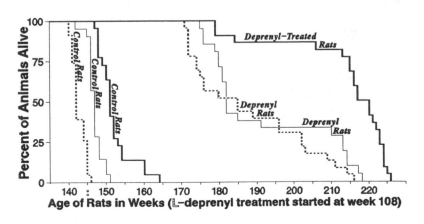

before the first of the deprenyl-treated rats had died. Data from three groups of rats are displayed. The broken line represents the rats no longer exhibiting any sexual activity, the thin line represents the rats still exhibiting some sexual activity, and the bold line represents rats still able to sexually function (although not necessarily well). The higher sexed rats generally lived longer, in both the deprenyl and control groups.

Some conservative people will want to wait until deprenyl's life-extending effects are proven on humans before they take it themselves. If such studies are initiated, everyone waiting for the results will be long dead before the study is ever completed. Our guess (and the guess of most people familiar with the research) is that deprenyl will do exactly the same thing to humans that it does to animals — slow down aging. This is why many people we know (including the authors) are taking deprenyl.

Deprenyl for Alzheimer's Disease

Deprenyl has become a powerful new weapon against Alzheimer's disease. In a study in Italy, 10 Alzheimer's patients were given either a placebo or 5 mg of deprenyl twice a day for two months. The results showed that deprenyl improved memory, attention, and language abilities among those who received the drug, while those who received placebo became worse [Agnoli, *et al.*, 1992]. Another study of 20 Alzheimer's patients treated with deprenyl for six months also showed significant improvements in memory and attention [Piccinin, *et al.*, 1990].

Verbal memory was tested in patients with Alzheimer's disease in yet another double-blind randomized crossover trial which also lasted 6 months. Each subject was tested before, during, and after the study with the Rey-Auditory-Verbal Learning Test. Deprenyl brought about a significant improvement in verbal memory, and "improved information processing abilities and learning strategies at the moment of acquisition" [Finali, *et al.*, 1992].

Numerous other studies have shown similar positive results in people with Alzheimer's disease [Goad, *et al.*, 1991; Finali, *et al.*, 1991; Sloane, 1991; Mangoni, *et al.*, 1991; Martini, *et al.*, 1987].

Dr. Knoll [1992] states bluntly that "Alzheimer's disease patients need to be treated daily with 10 mg deprenyl from diagnosis until death." See our Suggested Treatment Protocols chapter for specifics on the use of deprenyl for people with Alzheimer's disease.

Deprenyl Versus Other Drugs for Alzheimer's Disease

Oxiracetam (a nootropic drug similar to piracetam — see the chapter on oxiracetam in Smart Drugs & Nutrients) was tested against deprenyl in a trial involving 22 men and 18 women with mild-to-moderate Alzheimer's disease. Ten milligrams per day of deprenyl were given to one group and 800 mg per day of oxiracetam were given to the other group. The results showed that at these doses, deprenyl was more effective than oxiracetam in improving higher cognitive functions and reducing impairment in daily living. Deprenyl helped more with short- and long-term memory, sustained concentration, attention, verbal fluency, and visuospatial abilities. Both drugs were well tolerated with few or no side effects [Falsaperla, *et al.*, 1990].

In another study, deprenyl was compared to phosphatidylserine in forty people with Alzheimer's disease. The dosage of deprenyl was 10 mg per day and that of phosphatidylserine was 200 mg per day. Both treatments lasted three months. For most measures of cognition, the deprenyl group did better [Monteverde, *et al.*, 1990]. (See the Phosphatidylserine chapter in this book.)

Deprenyl was also compared to acetyl-L-carnitine (ALC) in forty people with mild-to-moderate Alzheimer's disease. Deprenyl (10 mg per day) was slightly more effective than ALC (500 mg twice daily), but we believe that the dosage of ALC may have been too low. However, it is interesting that both drugs were effective [Campi, *et al.*, 1990]. (See the Acetyl-L-Carnitine Update chapter.)

Deprenyl Improves Cognition in Parkinson's Disease

Deprenyl is becoming recognized as the treatment of choice for people with Parkinson's disease. Although it is well known that deprenyl dramatically slows down the progression of the disease, it is not so widely recognized that deprenyl also improves cognition in people with Parkinsonism. Several studies show that deprenyl improves attention, memory, and reaction times in Parkinson's patients. It also brings about subjective feelings of increased vitality, euphoria, and increased energy [Lees, 1991].

Deprenyl significantly delays the progression of Parkinson's disease under many conditions. Newly-diagnosed patients treated with deprenyl take far longer for their symptoms to become bad enough to require L-dopa (L-dopa used to be the drug of choice for Parkinson's disease). Many patients on deprenyl never require L-dopa. In addition, advanced Parkinson's patients treated with deprenyl plus L-dopa live longer than those treated with L-dopa alone.

Better Than Chocolate

Deprenyl is chemically related to phenylethylamine (PEA), a substance found in chocolate and produced in higher-than-normal amounts in the brains of people who are "in love." Deprenyl's chemical structure is also closely related to amphetamine which, like PEA, is able to cross into brain neurons and trigger the release of the neurotransmitters norepinephrine, epinephrine and dopamine. The release of these neurotransmitters causes mental stimulation and increased alertness.

Deprenyl, however, does not trigger neurotransmitter release. In this respect, deprenyl is unique among PEA derivatives.

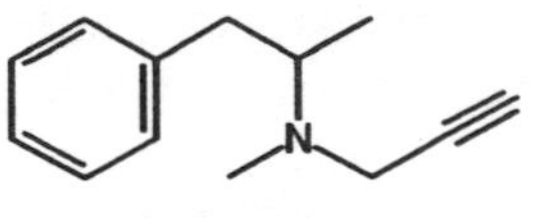

L-Deprenyl
(selegiline)

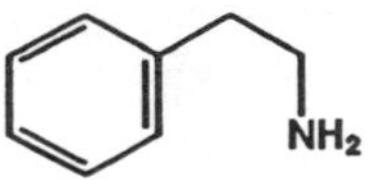

PEA
(phenethylamine)

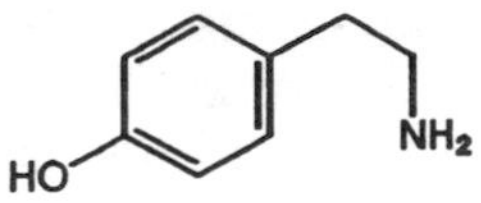

Tyramine

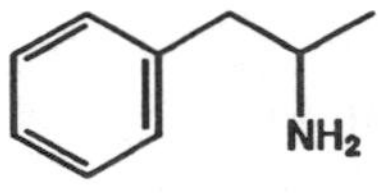

Amphetamine

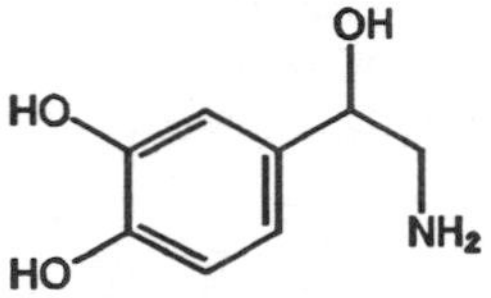

Norepinephrine

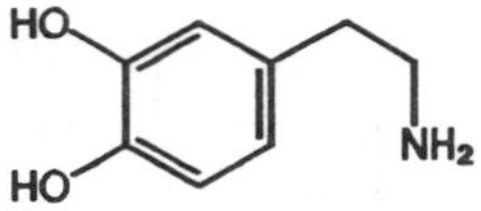

Dopamine

Deprenyl is a member of a class of drugs called monoamine oxidase (MAO) inhibitors. MAO is an enzyme responsible for breaking down used neurotransmitters so that they can be excreted. MAO levels tend to rise with age, and as a result, brain levels of monoamine neurotransmitters like dopamine tend to fall with age.

MAO inhibition can correct this age-related decrease in neurotransmitters. However, when MAO is over-inhibited, neurotransmitters can build up to excessive levels causing neuronal hyperstimulation — hence the 'speediness' effect of amphetamines. Deprenyl manages to avoid this side effect by inhibiting only a selected form of MAO.

Forms of Monoamine Oxidase

MAO enzymes are found throughout the body and come in two known types: type A (found in most body tissues), and type B (found predominantly in brain glial cells). Glial cells are small brain cells which surround and metabolically support the neurons which conduct the electrical signals throughout the brain.

Most MAO inhibitors are unselective, inhibiting both MAO-A and MAO-B to a similar degree. When MAO-A is inhibited (as with amphetamines, for example), a dangerous high-blood-pressure reaction can occur in patients who eat certain foods like aged cheeses, chianti wines, and chicken liver paté, which contain a chemical called tyramine. Tyramine is usually metabolized by MAO, and inhibition of MAO causes tyramine to dangerously accumulate. This same high-blood-pressure reaction can occur in patients taking L-dopa for Parkinson's disease. Unlike other MAO inhibitors, however, deprenyl inhibits only MAO-B. It does not cause the "cheese reaction" and it can be safely administered with L-dopa.

Deprenyl was the first selective MAO-B inhibitor to be described in the scientific literature. Over the last 30 years, it has become the reference standard for MAO-B inhibition. It is still the only one in widespread clinical use today.

How Does it Work?

Deprenyl is the only drug known to selectively enhance the activity of a tiny region of the brain called the substantia nigra. The substantia nigra is exceptionally rich in dopaminergic (dopamine-using) neurons. Dopamine is the neurotransmitter that regulates such primitive functions as motor control and sex drive. Deficiencies of dopamine result in Parkinson's disease symptoms.

Degeneration of the neurons in the substantia nigra is implicated not only in the development of Parkinson's disease, but also in the aging process itself. Deprenyl protects against the age-related degeneration of the substantia nigra and dopaminergic nervous system. It also protects sensitive dopamine-containing neurons from age-associated increases in glial cells and the MAO-B that they contain.

Deprenyl also inhibits the degrading of neurotransmitters and boosts the release of dopamine. Deprenyl-induced enhancement of brain function manifests in several dramatic ways. Dopamine is crucial to sex-drive, fine motor control, immune function and motivation. The steep decline of dopamine-containing neurons in the human brain after age 45 is a universal characteristic of the aging process. The tiny substantia nigra region of the brain is richest in dopamine and undergoes the most rapid aging of any brain area. It is the *premature* aging of this region which causes Parkinson's disease. On the other hand, normal age-associated depletion of dopamine accounts for many other symptoms — most notably the gradual decline of male (and, possibly, female) sex drive.

Variable Aging in the Brain

The rate at which the dopamine neurons age is quite variable. Prior to age 40-45, dopamine levels remain fairly stable. Starting at age 40-45, average dopamine content in healthy individuals decreases by about 13% per decade (see illustration below). When it reaches approximately 30% of youthful levels (gray area), Parkinson's symptoms result. Below 10%, death results.

Those with average or slow decline die of other causes before Parkinson's symptoms become apparent. In fact, it has been suggested that if we all lived long enough, we would all eventually develop Parkinson's disease. As average and maximum lifespan is increased, the use of deprenyl will become even more critical for the prevention of dopamine-deficiency degenerative diseases. Treatment with deprenyl may come to be a central strategy in geriatrics.

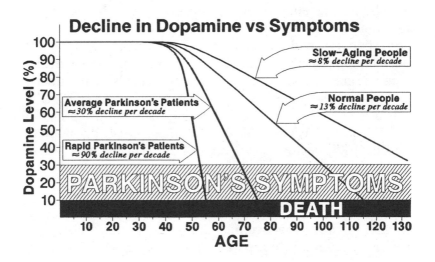

Dopamine activity in the brain is also increased by acetyl-L-carnitine (see the Acetyl-L-carnitine Update chapter).

Deprenyl for Depression

Deprenyl alone, or combined with phenylalanine, is often very effective at relieving depression. Phenylalanine is an amino acid that acts as a precursor (a chemical building block) to neurotransmitters such as norepinephrine.

In 1984, in Vienna, Dr. Birkmayer and colleagues treated 155 patients (102 outpatients and 53 inpatients) who were suffering from unipolar depression. The patients were given 5-10 mg of deprenyl and 250 mg of L-phenylalanine per day. The outpatients were treated orally, and 68.5% achieved "full remission." Of the remaining patients, 21.5% achieved "moderate improvement," 6% were unchanged, and 4% dropped out.

The inpatients were treated intravenously. Of these, 69.5% achieved full remission, 11% exhibited mild to moderate improvement, 12% showed no improvement and 7.5% dropped out. The therapeutic effect started one to three weeks into the treatment.

The beneficial effect of the daily intravenous infusion was maintained when the dose was reduced to twice a week, and also when switched to oral dosing. The authors noted that the outstanding clinical efficacy of deprenyl-plus-phenylalanine for depression was equaled only by electroconvulsive treatments (ECT) — without the memory-loss side effect of ECT. The side effects of the deprenyl-plus-phenylalanine were primarily sleeplessness, anxiety, and tension (these could probably be eliminated by decreasing the dose of phenylalanine, or adding a serotonergic precursor like tryptophan). The treatment was well tolerated in 90% of the patients, and no withdrawal symptoms were noted in any of the patients.

In another study conducted in Chicago, 6 out of ten patients suffering from "drug-resistant major depressive disorders" considered their depression totally relieved after only 2-3 days treatment with 5 mg of deprenyl, 100 mg of vitamin B_6, and 1-6 grams of phenylalanine per day. Their Global Assessment Scale scores dropped by 33% and stayed down over the remaining 6 weeks of the study [Sabelli, 1991]. The patients had been suffering from numerous depressions including manic depression, bipolar type II depression, schizoaffective disorder, seasonal affective disorder, and unipolar recurrent depression. Further double-blind research is underway.

The relatively slow response in the first study and fast response in the later study is probably due to the difference in phenylalanine dosage (250 mg vs. 1000-6000 mg respectively).

Conclusion

Deprenyl's low level of toxicity, few side effects, and uniquely broad spectrum of pharmacological activities make it ideal for protection against brain aging and the age-related decline of the dopaminergic nervous system. Deprenyl is the drug of choice for Parkinson's disease and is currently being established as a treatment for Alzheimer's disease. Eventually, deprenyl may become recognized as a general preventive treatment for aging and age-related degenerative diseases in the above-45-year-old population.

Precautions

Deprenyl is very safe. No mutation-causing or birth defect-causing effects have been observed with deprenyl. In animal experiments, the LD-50 (lethal) dose is approximately 300-500 times greater than the dose required for complete MAO-B inhibition. Human patients have tolerated up to 60 mg of deprenyl per day for over three weeks without difficulty. The hypertensive reaction that occurs with MAO-A inhibitors following ingestion of tyramine-containing foods (like cheese, chianti wine, beans, chicken liver) has not been observed in patients taking the standard 5-10 mg dose of deprenyl. This response is observed to some degree at the 60 mg dose.

Dosage

For Parkinsonism, the recommended dosage of deprenyl is 5-10 mg daily. For the healthy population 45 and older, Dr. Knoll recommends 10-15 mg per week. For 45-year-olds, we think this dose may be high. For younger people, much smaller doses may suffice. Some people take only $\frac{1}{4}$-$\frac{1}{2}$ tablet (1.25-2.5 mg) once a week. One manufacturer of deprenyl, Discovery Experimental and Development, recommends a more gradual, age- related dosing schedule which takes full advantage of their 1-mg-per-drop liquid deprenyl (see following table).

Recommended Deprenyl Dosages

Age	Dosage	Age	Dosage
30-35	1 mg twice a week	60-65	5 mg every day
35-40	1 mg every other day	65-70	6 mg every day
40-45	1 mg every day	70-75	8 mg every day
45-50	2 mg every day	75-80	9 mg every day
50-55	3 mg every day	80+	10 mg every day
55-60	4 mg every day		

Deprenyl causes a general stimulation of mental function that is distinctly different from that of other nutrients and drugs (phenylalanine, tyrosine, L-dopa, and amphetamine). Most people report a mild-to-moderate anti-depressant effect, increased energy, improved feelings of well-being, substantially increased sex drive, and more assertiveness. The effect is mild in low doses and can last for several days.

As the dose of deprenyl is increased, symptoms of overstimulation can result. People have reported feeling "over-amped," sexually overstimulated, nauseous, irritable, emotionally hyper-reactive, and even "detached" from their surroundings. When too much deprenyl is taken, the stimulation that it produces becomes L-dopa-like or amphetamine-like which can become tiresome because it lasts so long. At high doses, many people report such sleeping disturbances as vivid dreams, nightmares and insomnia.

With deprenyl, more is not necessarily better. As with most smart drugs, starting with low doses and increasing gradually is the best policy. When combining smart drugs you may need to reduce the dosages.

Sources

Also called l-deprenyl, L-deprenyl, (–)deprenyl, selegiline, Jumex, or Eldepryl, deprenyl is available throughout the world. As Eldepryl, deprenyl is available from any pharmacy in the U.S. or Canada with a physician's prescription. It is also available from a number of overseas mail-order pharmacies. You can obtain a list of such sources by mailing the tearout card at the front of this book to CERI (the Cognitive Enhancement Research Institute). CERI also publishes *Smart Drug News* which frequently includes information of interest to people who are using (or want to use) deprenyl.

A high purity liquid deprenyl manufactured by the Discovery Experimental and Development company (Wesley Chapel, Florida) has been submitted for approval by the FDA. It is already approved and available in Mexico. Discovery's liquid deprenyl has the added convenience of being dispensable in single milligram doses (1 mg per drop) as opposed to the standard 5 mg tablet. This makes it easier for healthy 40-50 year olds to take the correct amount (see the Dosage section in this chapter.)

References

Agnoli A, Fabbrini G, Fioravanti M and Martucci N. CBF and cognitive evaluation of Alzheimer type patients before and after MAO-B treatment: a pilot study. *Eur Neuropsychopharmacol* (Netherlands) 2(1): 31-5, March 1992.

Birkmayer W, Riederer P, Linauer W and Knoll J. L-Deprenyl plus L-phenylalanine in the treatment of depression. *Journal of Neural Transmission* 59: 81-7, 1984.

Brandeis R, Sapir M, Kapon Y, Borelli G, Cadel S and Valsecchi B. Improvement of cognitive function by MAO-B inhibitor L-deprenyl in aged rats. *Pharmacol Biochem Behav* (USA) 39(2): 297-304, 1991.

Campi N, Todeschini GP and Scarzella L. Selegiline versus L-acetylcarnitine in the treatment of Alzheimer-type dementia. *Clin Ther* 12(4): 306-14, Jul-Aug 1990.

Deprenyl

Carillo MC, Kanai S, Nohubo M, *et al.* (–)-Deprenyl induced activities of both superoxide dismutase and catalase in young male rats. *Life Sci* 48: 517, 1991.

Falsaperla A, Monici Preti PA and Oliani C. Selegiline versus oxiracetam in patients with Alzheimer-type dementia. *Clin Ther* 12(5): 376-84, Sep-Oct 1990.

Finali G, Piccirilli M, Oliani C and Piccinin GL. Alzheimer-type dementia and verbal memory performances: influence of selegiline therapy. *Ital J Neurol Sci* 13(2): 141-8, March 1992.

Finali G, Piccirilli M, Oliani C and Piccinin GL. L-deprenyl therapy improves verbal memory in amnesic Alzheimer patients. *Clin Neuropharmacol* (USA) 14(6): 523-36, 1991.

Goad DL, Davis CM, Liem P, Fuselier CC, McCormack JR and Olsen KM. The use of selegiline in Alzheimer's patients with behavior problems. *J Clin Psychiatry* 52(8): 342-5, August 1991. Also see comments, *J Clin Psychiatry* 53(3): 101-2, March 1992.

Knoll J. (–)Deprenyl-medication: A strategy to modulate the age-related decline of the striatal dopaminergic system. *J Am Geriatr Soc* 40(8): 839-47, August 1992.

Knoll J. Extension of lifespan of rats by long-term (–)deprenyl treatment. *Mount Sinai J Med* 55: 67-74, 1988.

Knoll J. Pharmacological basis of the therapeutic effect of (–)deprenyl in age-related neurological diseases. *Med Res Rev* (United States) 12(5): 505-24, September 1992.

Knoll J. Pharmacological basis of the therapeutic effect of (–)deprenyl in age-related neurological diseases. *Med Res Rev* (United States) 12(5): 505-24, Sept 1992.

Knoll J. The pharmacology of selegiline ((–)deprenyl). New aspects. *Acta Neurol. Scand.* 126: 83-91, 1989.

Knoll J. The pharmacology of selegiline (–)deprenyl: New aspects. *Acta Neurol Scand* 126: 83, 1989.

Knoll J. The possible mechanism of action of (–)deprenyl in Parkinson's disease. *Journal of Neural Transmission* 43: 239-44, 1978.

Knoll J. The striatal dopamine dependency of lifespan in male rats. Longevity study with (–)deprenyl. *Mechanisms of Aging and Development* 46: 237-62, 1988.

Knoll J, Yen TT and Dallo J. Long-lasting, true aphrodisiac effect of (–)deprenyl in sluggish old male rats. *Mod Probl Pharmacopsychiat* 19: 135-53, 1983.

Lees AJ. Selegiline hydrochloride and cognition. *Acta Neurol Scand Suppl* 136: 91-4, 1991.

Letters to the Editor on deprenyl in Parkinson's disease, *The New England Journal of Medicine* 322: 1526-7, 24 May 1990.

Mangoni A, Grassi MP, Frattola L, Piolti R, Bassi S, Motta A, Marcone A and Smirne S. Effects of a MAO-B inhibitor in the treatment of Alzheimer's disease. *Eur Neurol* (Switzerland) 31(2): 100-7, 1991.

Martini E, Pataky I, Szilagyi K and Venter V. Brief information on an early phase-II-study with deprenyl in demented patients. *Pharmacopsychiatry* (Germany, Federal Republic of) 20(6): 256-257, 1987.

Milgram NW, *et al.* Maintenance on L-deprenyl prolongs life in aged male rats. *Life Sciences* 47: 415-20, 1990.

Monteverde A, Gnemmi P, Rossi F, Monteverde A and Finali GC. Selegiline in the treatment of mild to moderate Alzheimer-type dementia. *Clin Ther* 12(4): 315-22, Jul-Aug 1990.

The Parkinson Study Group, Effect of deprenyl on the progression of disability in early Parkinson's disease. *The New England Journal of Medicine* 321: 1364-71, 16 November 1989.

Piccinin GL, Finali G and Piccirilli M. Neuropsychological effects of L-deprenyl in Alzheimer's type dementia. *Clin Neuropharmacol* 13(2): 147-63, April 1990.

Sabelli HC. Rapid treatment of depression with selegiline-phenylalanine combination. *Journal of Clinical Psychiatry* 53(3): 137, March 1991.

Schneider LS, Pollock VE, Zemansky MF, Gleason RP, Palmer R and Sloane RB. A pilot study of low-dose L-deprenyl in Alzheimer's disease. *J Geriatr Psychiatry Neurol* (USA) 4(3): 143-8, 1991.

Tariot PN, *et al.* L-Deprenyl in Alzheimer's disease: Preliminary evidence for behavioral change with monoamine oxidase B inhibition. *Archives of General Psychiatry* 44: 427-33, May 1987.

Deprenyl

Melatonin

The pineal gland, until recently, has been referred to as mystery gland, since its functions were largely unknown. The pineal is now recognized as a key element in the maintenance of the body's endocrine regulation (hormone balance), immune system integrity, and circadian rhythm (daily metabolic balance). Melatonin is the principal hormone produced by the pineal gland. Melatonin is under investigation as a treatment for a number of conditions, including jet-lag, seasonal affective disorder (SAD), depression, and cancer. Pineal polypeptide extract (which contains a broad spectrum of other, protein-based pineal hormones) has been shown to inhibit the development of atherosclerosis [Tasca, *et al.*, 1974], reduce blood triglyceride levels [Ostroumova and Vasiljeve, 1976], improve cellular immunity [Belokrylov, *et al.*, 1976; Dilman, 1977], and increase lifespan in animals [Dilman, *et al.*, 1979].

The pineal gland functions as a biological clock by secreting melatonin (along with many other neuropeptides) at night. As you can see from the following illustration, melatonin levels

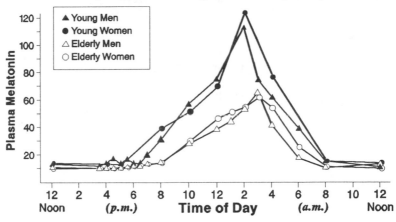

Melatonin Secretion in Young and Elderly People

peak at about 2 a.m. in normal, healthy young people and about 3 a.m. in elderly people. The maximum amount of melatonin released in the bloodstream of the elderly is only half of that in young adults.

Melatonin levels are low during the day. At sunset, the cessation of light triggers neural signals which stimulate the pineal gland to begin releasing melatonin. This rise continues for hours, eventually peaking around 2 a.m. (3 a.m. for the elderly) after which it steadily declines to minimal levels by morning. The delay in timing and decrease in intensity of the melatonin pulse is a manifestation of the aging process.

The melatonin pulse regulates many neuroendocrine functions. When the timing or intensity of the melatonin peak is disrupted (as in aging, stress, jet-lag, or artificial jet-lag syndromes), many

Age–Related Changes in Melatonin Levels

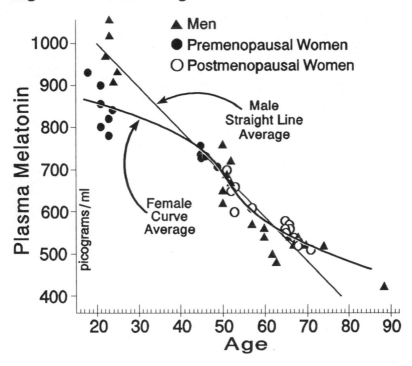

physiological and mental functions are adversely affected. The ability to think clearly, remember key facts, and make sound decisions can be profoundly hampered by these upsets in the biological clock.

Melatonin for Jet-Lag

Jet-lag is a condition caused by desynchronization of the biological clock. It is usually caused by drastically changing your sleep-wake cycle, as when crossing several time zones during east-west travel, or when performing shift work. Jet-lag is characterized by fatigue, early awakening or insomnia, headache, fuzzy thinking, irritability, constipation, and reduced immunity. The symptoms are generally worse when flying in an easterly direction, and it may take as long as one day for each time zone crossed in order to fully recover. Older people have an even tougher time adjusting to these changes than younger people.

Circadian disturbances can easily result from conditions other than jet travel. We call these "artificial jet-lag syndromes" because jet-lag is universally understood. Artificial jet-lag can be induced by working night shifts, working rotating shifts (like physician-interns, management trainees for 24-hour businesses, and soldiers under battle-alert conditions), or by staying up all

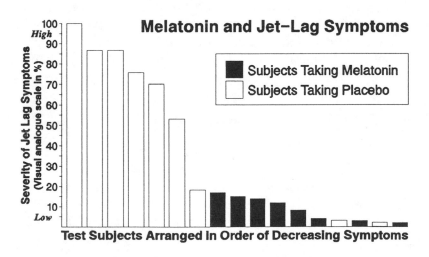

Melatonin and Jet–Lag Symptoms

Severity of Jet Lag Symptoms (Visual analogue scale in %)

■ Subjects Taking Melatonin
□ Subjects Taking Placebo

Test Subjects Arranged In Order of Decreasing Symptoms

night. Whatever its causes, jet-lag and artificial jet-lag syndromes are seriously debilitating to cognitive function.

Melatonin taken in the evening (in the new time zone!) will rapidly reset your biological clock and almost totally alleviate (or prevent) the symptoms of jet-lag. The ability of melatonin to alleviate jet-lag was demonstrated in a study of 17 subjects flying from San Francisco to London (eight time zones away). Eight subjects took 5 mg of melatonin, while nine subjects took a placebo. Those who took melatonin had almost no symptoms of jet-lag (see illustration below) [Arendt, *et al.*, 1986]. Six out of nine placebo subjects scored above 50 on the jet lag scale, and all of the melatonin subjects scored below 17.

Most people sleep well with melatonin, and wake up the next day refreshed with no symptoms of jet-lag [Claustrat, 1992] (although they may still have some fatigue from the wear and tear of traveling).

Many melatonin fans without any noticeable symptoms of circadian disturbance are now using melatonin to enhance their circadian rhythms. They report that it helps them get to sleep and helps them sleep more soundly. It also makes them more alert the next day and even lessens mid-afternoon tiredness (and naps).

In all cases, melatonin should be taken at night (preferably before midnight) before going to bed. That's when your pineal gland naturally releases melatonin. Taking melatonin at night (or before your normal bedtime if you are a shift worker) helps restore and maintain normal circadian metabolic rhythms. See the Precautions section in this chapter.

Does Melatonin Improve or Impair Mental Performance?

We were initially surprised to find a number of studies which reported on adverse effects of melatonin on performance and alertness. One study [Lieberman, 1984] reported that melatonin users were less alert, more sleepy, and demonstrated slowed "choice-reaction time." Other studies also indicated that melatonin impaired memory and performance [Neville, 1986]. We found, however, that in all of these studies, melatonin was given to subjects in the *daytime*, before the performance tests, just the opposite of what they should have been doing!

With circadian enhancers like melatonin, the timing is critical. When taken in opposition to the body's natural circadian rhythm, they cause cognitive deficit just like jet-lag does. But when taken in synchronization with the body's natural circadian rhythms, they enhance mental performance. By giving melatonin in the daytime, before the cognitive tests, the researchers were causing the test subjects to suffer from artificial jet-lag and then measuring the resulting cognitive impairment. Disruption of circadian rhythms produces amnesia by interfering with the circadian organization of memory processes [Sandyk, 1991].

Melatonin, by correcting circadian rhythms should, theoretically, improve mental performance. We could only find one study in which melatonin was given to rats at night. This study confirmed that next-day measures of learning ability improved [Ovanesov, 1990].

We believe that melatonin, when taken before sleep, will decrease sleep disturbances of any kind, and will, therefore, improve mental function during the following day.

Melatonin for SAD and Depression

Two particularly notable features of depression and SAD are diminished nighttime release of melatonin and abnormal sensitivity to melatonin suppression by light [Brown, 1989]. This has led researchers and clinicians to try melatonin as an experimental treatment for depression, with gratifying results.

Melatonin Extends Lifespan

Melatonin has also been shown to improve immunity and extend lifespan in rodents [Regelson & Pierpaoli, 1987; Pierpaoli, *et al.*, 1990]. Dr. Maestroni [1988] gave melatonin to middle-aged mice each evening. The treated mice became more healthy (better posture, increased activity levels, and thicker, more lustrous fur) and lived an average of 20% longer than control mice.

Melatonin secretion naturally drops off with age (see the following graph). This decrease is so reliable that blood melatonin levels have been proposed as a measurement of biological age [Nair, *et al.*, 1986]. This age-related reduction in melatonin levels may partially account for the reason many older people have difficulty sleeping at night, and for why they are so fatigued during the day. We believe they may be suffering from age-induced "jet-lag." Restoration of normal sleep-wake cycles in many of my [WD] elderly patients with supplemental melatonin before bedtime has dramatically improved their quality of life.

Melatonin: Anti-Stress Hormone

Nighttime administration of melatonin can also counteract the immune-suppressing effects of acute anxiety stress in mice. Measures used to confirm this were: thymus weight, antibody production, and ability to fight off a lethal viral infection [Pierpaoli and Maestroni, 1987].

Melatonin for Cancer Treatment

Melatonin also appears to inhibit tumor growth. In the United Kingdom, a study was carried out on 14 cancer patients with cancers of different types. The researchers concluded that "this study would suggest that melatonin may be of value in untreatable metastatic cancer patients, particularly in improving their quality of life. Moreover, based on its effects on the immune system, melatonin could be tested in association with other anti-tumor treatments" [Lissoni, 1989].

Melatonin in Alzheimer's Disease

Very recent studies have found reduced levels of melatonin in the cerebrospinal fluid of patients with Alzheimer's disease compared to age-matched control subjects [Tohgi, 1992; Skene, 1990]. Since circadian rhythms are disrupted in Alzheimer's disease, it is interesting to speculate whether restoration of melatonin to normal levels in these patients would alleviate other symptoms as well.

Melatonin and Exposure to Electromagnetic Fields

Sunlight is the primary environmental influence that regulates the internal clock and the associated late-night melatonin pulse. There is some evidence that the earth's magnetic field may also be an environmental signal affecting circadian rhythms in humans. When shielded from the earth's ambient magnetic field, human circadian rhythms can become disrupted [Tohgi, 1992].

Exposure to electromagnetic fields from appliances and from powerlines may be even more significant than we think. There are reports of altered neural function from exposure to ELF (extremely low frequency) fields, as found near high-voltage powerlines, including suppressed melatonin levels [Lovely, 1988]. Supplemental melatonin may help to overcome the negative health consequences of these fields.

Dosage

The appropriate dose can vary enormously from person to person. Dr. Pierpaoli, a leading melatonin researcher, has successfully used dosages ranging from 0.1 to 200 mg. That's a 2000-fold difference between the lowest dose and the highest! Several intelligent melatonin users we know started by taking 3 mg at 11 p.m., and then adjusted the dose from there. If they found that they slept well but were drowsy in the morning, they cut the dose in half. If they found the dose had little or no sleep-inducing effect, they increased the dose by 3 mg each night until they got the desired effect. We have received reports from one person who gets good results from less than one milligram, and several from people who use in the vicinity of 20 mg. Most people get good results with doses between 3 and 10 mg.

Precautions

Timing may be crucial for the most effective use of melatonin. Individual differences in the absorption and metabolism of melatonin may account for the differences in size and timing of the resulting melatonin pulse. A good illustration of this effect is found in the experiences of Dr. Tzischinsky [1992] of the medical university in Haifa, Israel. Dr. Tzischinsky treated an 18-year-old blind man suffering from chronic sleep disturbances. Presumably, the young man's blindness prevented sunlight from cueing his circadian rhythm. He suffered from daytime fatigue, often falling asleep during the day, but was awake at night. After two unsuccessful treatment regimens with 5 mg and 10 mg melatonin administered at bedtime (10 - 10:30 p.m.), Dr. Tzischinsky tried a third regimen of only 5 mg administered at 8 p.m. for three weeks. This approach resulted in a successful resolution of the man's sleep disturbances.

This observation (and others like it) demonstrate the importance of not only adjusting the dosage but also the time of the dose. Melatonin seems to be much more critical in this regard than other smart drugs. One melatonin user reports that he gave himself terrible jet-lag by absent-mindedly taking melatonin at 3 a.m. after staying up late. He recovered from this error, resetting his circadian rhythm back to normal with melatonin at 10 p.m. the following evening, but not before he had to spend an entire day in jet-lag hell for his mistake.

Sources

Melatonin is a non-prescription substance and can often be found where supplements are sold. For information about mail-order sources for melatonin you can send in the tearout card at the front of this book and ask for the product sources list. (See also Appendix A).

References

Arendt J, Aldhous M and Marks V. Alleviation of jet-lag by melatonin: Preliminary results of controlled double-blind trial. *Brit Med J* 292: 1170, 1986.

Belokrylov GA, Morozov VG, Khavinson VH, et al. The action of low molecular extracts from heterological thymus, pineal and hypothalamus on the immune response in mice. *Biull Eksp Biol Med* 81: 202-4, 1976.

Brown GM. Psychoneuroendocrinology of depression. *Psychiatr J Univ Ott* 14(2): 344-8; Jun 1989. Discussion follows article.

Claustrat B, Brun J, David M, Sassolas G and Chazot G. Melatonin and jet-lag: Confirmatory result using a simplified protocol. *Biol Psychiatry* (USA) 32(8): 705-11, 1992.

Dilman VM, Anisimov VN, and Ostroumova MN. Increase in lifespan of rats following polypeptide pineal extract treatment. *Exp Pathology* 17: 539-45, 1979.

Dilman VM. Improvement of cell-mediated immunity after pineal gland extract treatment. *Vopr Oncol* (Problems of Oncology) 7: 70-72, 1977.

Lieberman HR, Waldhauser F, Garfield G, et al. Effects of melatonin on human mood and performance. Brain Res (Netherlands) 323(2): 201-7, 1984.

Lissoni P, Barni S, Crispino S, Tancini G and Fraschini F. Endocrine and immune effects of melatonin therapy in metastatic cancer patients. *Eur J Cancer Clin Oncol* (United Kingdom) 25(5): 789-95, 1989.

Lovely RH. Recent studies in the behavioral toxicology of ELF electric and magnetic fields. *Prog Clin Biol Res* 257: 327-47, 1988.

Maestroni GJ, Conti A and Pierpaoli W. Pineal melatonin, its fundamental immuno-regulatory role in aging and cancer. *Ann N Y Acad Sci* 521: 140-8, 1988.

Maurizi CP. The therapeutic potential for tryptophan and melatonin: possible roles in depression, sleep, Alzheimer's disease and abnormal aging. *Med Hypotheses* 31(3): 233-42, March 1990.

Nair NPV, Hariharasubramanian N, Pilapil C, Issac I, and Thavundayil JX. Plasma melatonin — an index of brain aging in humans? *Biological Psychiatry* 21: 141-50, 1986.

Neville K and McNaughton N. Anxiolytic-like action of melatonin on acquisition but not performance of DRL. *Pharmacol Biochem Behav* 24(6): 1497-502, June 1986.

Ostroumova MN and Vasiljeve IA. Effect or polypeptide pineal extract on fat- carbo-hydrate metabolism. *Probl Endokrinol* 22: 66-9, 1976.

Ovanesov KB. Vliianie ostrogo i khronicheskogo vvedeniia melatonina na pereo-buchenie krys v U-obraznom labirinte i ikh chuvstvitel'nost' k galoperidolu [The effect of the acute and chronic administration of melatonin on the relearning of rats in a Y maze and their sensitivity to haloperidol]. *Farmakol Toksikol* 53(2): 15-7, Mar-Apr 1990.

Pierpaoli W, Changxian VI and Dall'aza A. Aging — Postponing effect of circadian melatonin: Experimental evidence, significance and possible mechanism. *Intern J Neuroscience* 51: 334-342, 1990.

Pierpaoli W and Maestroni GJM. Melatonin: A principal neuroimmunoregulatory and anti-stress hormone: Its anti-aging effects. *Immunol Lett* (Netherlands) 16(3-4): 355-61, 1987.

Regelson W and Pierpaoli W. Melatonin: a rediscovered antitumor hormone? *Cancer Investig* 5: 379-385, 1987.

Melatonin

Sandyk R, Anninos PA and Tsagas N. Age-related disruption of circadian rhythms: possible relationship to memory impairment and implications for therapy with magnetic fields. *Int J Neurosci* (England) 59(4): 259-62, Aug 1991.

Skene DJ, Vivien-Roels B, Sparks DL, Hunsaker JC, Pevet P, Ravid D and Swaab DF. Daily variation in the concentration of melatonin and 5-methoxytryptophol in the human pineal gland: effect of age and Alzheimer's disease. *Brain Res* 528(1): 170-4, 24 Sept 1990.

Souetre E, Salvati E, Krebs B, Belugou JL and Darcourt G. Abnormal melatonin response to 5-methoxypsoralen in dementia. *Am J Psychiatry* 146(8): 1037-40, Aug 1989.

Tasca C, Damian E and Stefaneanu L. Disappearance of aortic lesions in the rabbits with experimental atheromatosis after pineal extraction administration. *Rev Roum d'Endocr* 11: 209-13, 1974.

Tohgi H, Abe T, Takahashi S, Kimura M, Takahashi J and Kikuchi T. Concentrations of serotonin and its related substances in the cerebrospinal fluid in patients with Alzheimer-type dementia. *Neurosci Lett* (Ireland) 141(1): 9-12, 1992.

Tzischinsky O, Pal I, Epstein R, Dagan Y and Lavie P. The importance of timing in melatonin administration in a blind man. *J Pineal Res* (Denmark) 12(3): 105-8, 1992.

Milacemide

Late in 1991, newspapers, wire services, and television networks reported scientific findings on milacemide, claiming it to be the *first* drug to improve memory retrieval in normal, healthy humans. Milacemide does improve memory in normal, healthy humans but it is hardly the first drug to do so. Nevertheless, it is refreshing to see the mainstream media accord this smart-drug research its fifteen minutes of fame.

Memory Effects

In numerous studies, milacemide (2-n-pentylaminoacetamide) has been shown to improve human selective attention, word retrieval, numeric memory, and vigilance.

In one study, conducted by Dr. Barbara L. Schwartz [1991], milacemide enhanced the speed and accuracy of word retrieval from long-term memory in healthy humans. Sixty-four healthy subjects participated in the study, split evenly between men and women, young and old, and milacemide and placebo. Enhanced word-retrieval abilities were noted in both young (age 19-34) and old (age 60-78) subjects.

Milacemide's effect was found to be selective. Source memory (memory of the context in which a fact was learned) was significantly improved, whereas item memory (memory of the fact itself), was not. In young subjects, source memory accuracy increased from 74% to 79% correct. In older subjects, scores increased from 75% to 84% correct among milacemide users.

Milacemide readily crosses the blood-brain barrier where it is converted to glycinamide (by monoamine oxidase B) and then to glycine. Glycine is the smallest of the amino acids and also an excitatory neurotransmitter. It interacts with brain receptors known to be involved with the long-term potentiation of memory.

milacemide   *glycinamide*   *glycine*

Potentiation of NMDA Receptors

Recent research into learning and memory has pointed to the essential role of the N-methyl-D-aspartate (NMDA) receptor complex. NMDA receptors are critical for the induction of long-term potentiation of memory, a term which refers to the lasting power of memories. Glycine acts on the NMDA receptor complex to potentiate NMDA activity. Experimentally, compounds which enhance NMDA activity also enhance learning, while compounds which impair NMDA function also impair learning. In animals, milacemide has been found to reverse drug-induced impairment of memory.

Researchers are interested in milacemide because glycine itself cannot readily cross the blood-brain barrier. To raise glycine concentrations above "normal," glycine must be bound within a larger molecule (like milacemide), which can be absorbed into the brain (like a molecular Trojan horse) and subsequently broken down to release glycine. If milacemide proves clinically useful, other glycine-containing drugs may be developed.

Alzheimer's Disease Findings

Unfortunately, milacemide's effects on cognitive function have not been confirmed in Alzheimer's patients. In a double-blind, placebo-controlled study of over 200 men and women with Alzheimer's disease, conducted by Dr. Maurice W. Dysken and colleagues [1992], no cognitive benefit was observed during one month of treatment. Longer-term results from milacemide in Alzheimer's disease have not yet been published.

Milacemide has likewise shown no therapeutic effect in the treatment of schizophrenia [Rosse, 1990, 1991]. This puts milacemide in legal limbo. It appears to be useful only for memory enhancement in *normal, healthy people*. Unfortunately, the FDA currently will only approve drugs for the treatment of diseases, not for what they consider a normal condition. Thus, milacemide, and possibly all future glycine-containing drugs which may also be found to display the unfortunate property of improving cognitive function in normal persons but not in those with cognitive disorders, may languish on laboratory shelves due to FDA's Catch-22 policies.

Milacemide is manufactured by the pharmaceutical giant, Searle, which funded much of the research. Searle spokesperson Debbie Santy commented that, "With the growing aging population of the country, any possible treatment for age-associated illnesses will be in great demand." Unfortunately, age-associated memory impairment is not yet a recognized illness. Searle may be stuck with a great drug for which there is a huge demand and which they can't legally sell.

Precautions

Milacemide appears to have minimal toxicity. Of 115 patients in the above-mentioned Alzheimer's study, only four experienced elevated liver enzymes and had to drop out of the study. Two other milacemide patients dropped out of the study for other reasons (one for nausea and diarrhea, and the other for hospitalization due to disorientation). This incidence exactly matched the two control patients who dropped out (one for myocardial ischemia, and the other for a spontaneous bone fracture). With the noted exception of increased liver enzyme levels, milacemide was well tolerated.

Because milacemide is metabolized to glycinamide by MAO-B, MAO-B inhibitors may counteract the cognitive benefits of milacemide. Indeed, in rats, milacemide combined with deprenyl (an irreversible MAO-B inhibitor) or RO 16-6941 (a reversible MAO-B inhibitor) produced dramatic *negative synergy* in learning and avoidance behavior tests. This means the combination made the rats dumber than they were without the drugs! The negative synergy may be the result of accumulated unmetabolized milacemide which may have some kind of direct neurotoxicity.

▷ WARNING: Do not use milacemide in combination with any MAO-B inhibitor such as deprenyl.

Dosage

Milacemide has a strong inverted-U-shaped dose-response curve. While 10 mg/kg doses produce significant improvement in both passive and active avoidance learning in mice, the 3 mg/kg and 30 mg/kg doses provided no improvement and may have caused impairment of learning. This correlates well with the 400-1200 mg daily dosages found to increase mental performance in humans. When combining smart drugs you may need to reduce the dosages.

Sources

We do not yet know where to get milacemide, but if a source turns up, you can find out as soon as we do by staying in touch with CERI, the publishers of *Smart Drug News*. You can send in the tearout card at the front of this book for CERI's current product sources list.

Magnesium glycinate is available in health food stores under different brand names. One very reliable, high-quality mail-order source for it is Klaire Laboratories (see Appendix A).

Future Outlook

Despite negative synergy with deprenyl and other MAO-B inhibitors, milacemide shows clear evidence of cognitive enhancement in normal, healthy humans. In the future, perhaps other glycine-delivery drugs will be developed which will not require metabolism by MAO-B.

References

Dysken MW, *et al*. Milacemide: a placebo-controlled study in senile dementia of the Alzheimer type. *Journal of the American Geriatrics Society* 40: 503-6, 1992.

Handelmann GE, *et al*. Milacemide, a glycine pro-drug, enhances performance of learning tasks in normal and amnestic rodents. *Pharmacology Biochemistry and Behavior* 34: 823-28, 1989.

Quartermain D, *et al*. Milacemide enhances memory storage and alleviates spontaneous forgetting in mice. *Pharmacology Biochemistry and Behavior* 39: 31-5, 1991.

Rosse RB, *et al*. An open-label trial of milacemide in schizophrenia: an NMDA intervention strategy. *Clinical Neuropharmacology* 13(4): 348-54, 1990.

Rosse RB, *et al*. An NMDA intervention strategy in schizophrenia with "low-dose" milacemide. *Clinical Neuropharmacology* 14(3): 268-72, 1991.

Saletu B and Grünberger J. Early clinical pharmacological trials with a new anti-epileptic, milacemide, using pharmaco-EEG and psychometry. *Methods Find Exp Clin Pharmacol* 6: 317-30, 1984.

Saletu B, Grünberger J and Linzmayer L. Acute and subacute CNS effects of milacemide in elderly people: double-blind, placebo-controlled quantitative EEG and psychometric investigations. *Archives of Gerontology and Geriatrics* 5: 165-81, 1986.

Schwartz BL, *et al*. Glycine prodrug facilitates word retrieval in humans. *Neurology* 41: 1341-3, 1991.

Schwartz BL, *et al.*. The effects of milacemide on item and source memory. *Clinical Neuropharmacology* 15(2): 114-9, 1992.

Milacemide

Nimodipine

Kurt Z. Itil, Ph.D., President of HZI Research Center, Tarry-town, New York, sent us a very nice letter after reading *Smart Drugs & Nutrients*. He thought it was a fairly comprehensive book, but was surprised that we missed *nimodipine* in our research. Now that we've looked into it, we're surprised, too. Nimodipine is remarkable for the breadth of its effects. Along with deprenyl, pregnenolone, and acetyl-L-carnitine, nimodipine is one of the most promising substances being tested for the treatment of Alzheimer's disease. It's a memory enhancer in people with age-associated memory impairment, and also seems to have profound anti-stress and anti-aging benefits.

Nimodipine (Nimotop) is a member of a class of drugs known as calcium-channel blockers. Drugs in this class alter the flow of calcium ions through cell membranes. Calcium regulation is especially important for blood vessels and neurons, particularly those in the brain. Calcium-channel blockers are effective in a number of clinical conditions, including high blood pressure, migraine headaches, angina pectoris, and congestive heart failure. One of the effects of nimodipine is to increase blood flow in the brain by preventing constriction of cerebral blood vessels, principally those with the smallest diameters. Nimodipine also appears to increase acetylcholine levels.

As with many of the smart drugs we've discussed, nimodipine's FDA-approved use is not the one we are most interested in. Miles Pharmaceuticals received U.S. approval in 1989 to market nimodipine for treatment of hemorrhagic stroke. Nimodipine "improves the neurological outcome in these patients by reducing the incidence and severity of ischemic deficits" (meaning it improves blood flow in the brain and lessens oxygen deprivation). But, as one researcher stated, "the therapeutic usefulness of nimodipine appears not to be limited to cerebral ischemia, but may include dementia, age-related degenerative diseases, epilepsy, and ethanol intoxication [Scriabine, 1989]."

Nimodipine to Treat Age-Associated Memory Impairment

Researchers in Italy conducted a long-term study to find out how nimodipine would affect the rate of "brain aging." They administered 90 mg of nimodipine each day to 40 patients between 65 and 80 years old suffering minor to medium signs of mental aging. An incredible 69.5% of the subjects showed improved mental performance as measured with a variety of mental tests. Twenty percent of the subjects did not change, and 9.5% worsened slightly. Remember that subjects of this age group would normally be expected to deteriorate to varying degrees over a six-month period. However, in this study, almost 70% of the subjects actually *improved* [Centonze, *et al.*, 1992].

Many other studies show that nimodipine is effective in improving memory in normal, healthy-but-aging animals [Scriabine, *et al.*, 1989; Levere, *et al.*, 1992; Straube, *et al.*, 1990; Sandin, *et al.*, 1990; Deyo, *et al.*, 1989; Isaacson, *et al.*, 1988; Schmage, *et al.*, 1992].

Nimodipine Improves Memories in Young Rats

One study we found tested the effects of nimodipine in young, healthy rats. This study showed that the treated rats learned more quickly than those which were not treated. The researchers also confirmed that nimodipine increased levels of acetylcholine in the hippocampus [Levy, *et al.*, 1991]. Although we have not yet seen any studies on memory improvement in young humans with nimodipine, we would expect the results to be positive, based on the compelling evidence cited above.

Nimodipine Reduces Stress-Related Consequences

Older female rats were given nimodipine and then submitted to a psychological stress-inducing situation. Untreated rats subjected to the same stressful conditions lost body weight, and some died. These adverse effects were not seen in those treated with nimodipine. The researchers concluded that nimodipine has a protective effect in stress-related illnesses [De Marino, et al., 1991].

Nimodipine for Treatment of Alzheimer's Disease

In 1990, one study showed that nimodipine was effective in the treatment of Alzheimer's disease. This was a 12-week, placebo-controlled, double-blind, multi-center study of 227 people with Alzheimer's disease. The people who received nimodipine were stabilized, while those who received placebo continued to decline [Tollefson, 1990].

Nimodipine for Old-Age Dementia

Researchers from Vanderbilt University in Nashville, Tennessee, conducted a multi-center, placebo-controlled, double-blind clinical study of 178 elderly patients with cognitive decline. Subjects were given either a placebo or 90 mg of nimodipine per day orally (30 mg three times daily). The study, which lasted 12 weeks, showed that nimodipine was effective in improving memory, depression, and general state of mind in these patients. There were only a few mild adverse effects noted during the 12 weeks of treatment [Ban, et al., 1990].

In the Netherlands, a one-year study was conducted to evaluate the effect of nimodipine in 20 patients with senile dementia. Half of the subjects lived in a nursing home, and the other half at home. Subjects were given a battery of tests every three months. Those who lived at home improved significantly, while those in the institutions showed only partial improvement. No adverse effects were noticed [Schinco, 1991].

Another recent study in China tested nimodipine on 46 patients with cerebrovascular disease. This double-blind study used either nimodipine or placebo. This study also showed an improvement in memory [Xu and Guo, 1991].

Other Effects of Nimodipine

Other uses of nimodipine include treatment for stroke, migraine and cluster headache, epilepsy, and anxiety.

Migraine headaches initially involve vasoconstriction, where the tiny blood vessels in the brain constrict. This is followed by a vasodilation phase. The headache is thought to occur during the cerebral vasodilation phase. Calcium-channel blockers such as nimodipine prevent the initial vasoconstriction *and* the following vasodilation phase.

Nimodipine also has anti-anxiety effects in animals and humans and changes EEG patterns in humans in the same way that other anti-anxiety drugs do [Langley, *et al.*, 1989; Itil, *et al.*, 1984; Itil, *et al.*, 1985; Hoffmeister, *et al.*, 1982].

Nimodipine has had an anti-convulsant effect in a few patients with a particular type of epilepsy called Koshevnikoff's epilepsy (or chronic focal epilepsy) [Brandt, *et al.*, 1988]. In animals, nimodipine prevents seizures induced by ischemia (oxygen deprivation), reperfusion (oxygen re-delivery after deprivation), or drugs [Meyer, 1986; Morocutti, *et al.*, 1986; Hoffmeister, *et al.*, 1982].

Also, in rats, nimodipine prevented seizures caused by withdrawal from chronic alcohol consumption [Little, *et al.*, 1986], and also reduced the symptoms of opiate withdrawal [Bongianni, *et al.*, 1986].

By blocking calcium channels on nerve cell membranes, nimodipine slows the entry of calcium into those cells. This has the effect of increasing the magnesium/calcium ratio. Would a magnesium supplement have some of the effects of nimodipine? Maybe. See the Vitamin Update chapter for further discussion of this possiblity.

Precautions

Nimodipine is generally well tolerated following oral adminis-tration. Adverse effects occurred in about 11% of the patients who received oral nimodipine in doses ranging from 30 mg to 120 mg (a very large dose) every four hours for the management of subarachnoid hemorrhage. Rarely reported adverse effects include: decreased blood pressure, abnormal liver function tests, edema, diarrhea, rash, headache, gastrointestinal symptoms, nausea, dyspnea (breathing difficulties), EKG abnormalities, tachycardia, bradycardia, muscle pain/cramp, acne, and depression.

➪ Safety and efficacy of nimodipine in children younger than 18 years of age have not been established. Nimodipine should not be used during pregnancy unless specified by a physician. This list is compiled from the *Physician's Desk Reference* and does not include adverse effects that occurred in less than 1% of subjects. Please read the *PDR* on this drug before using it.

➪ Nimodipine should not be used in conjunction with other calcium-channel blockers.

➪ Use of nimodipine with high doses of Dilantin (phenytoin) should be done only under a physician's care. This should involve frequent tests for plasma phenytoin concentrations.

Dosage

For treatment of subarachnoid hemorrhage, a dosage of 60 mg of nimodipine every four hours for 21 consecutive days is recommended. Dosages used in the above-mentioned studies on Alzheimer's disease used 90 mg per day (30 mg three times daily). For cognition-enhancement purposes in otherwise healthy individuals it may be best to start with a small fraction of the normal 30 mg capsule or tablet. When combining smart drugs you may need to reduce the dosages.

Sources

Nimodipine is a prescription drug in the U.S. Other names include Nimotop and Periplum. You can purchase it from a pharmacy if you have a doctor's prescription. For a listing of other sources, send in the tearout card at the front of this book. Some of the overseas sources for nimodipine have prices far lower than the standard U.S. retail price (see Appendix A for a listing of product sources).

References

Ban TA, et al.. Nimodipine in the treatment of old age dementias. Prog Neuropsychopharmacol Biol Psychiatry 14(4): 525-51, 1990.

Bongianni F, Carla V and Moroni F. Calcium channel inhibitors suppress the morphine-withdrawal syndrome in rats. Br J Pharmacol 88: 561-7, 1986.

Bower B. Boosting memory in the blink of an eye. Science News 135: p86, 11 February 1989.

Brandt L, Andersson KE, Ljunggren B, et al.. Cerebrovascular and cerebral effects of nimodipine — an update. Acta Neurochir 45(Suppl): 11-20, 1988.

Brandt L, Saveland H, Ljunggren B, et al.. Control of epilepsy partialis continuans with intravenous nimodipine. J Neurosurg 69: 949-50, 1988.

Centonze V, Massaro C, Polito BM, Cassiano MA, Di Bari M, Russo P, Cirillo L and Albano O. Invecchiamento cerebrale e farmaci calcio-antagonisti. Studio preliminare in aperto con la nimodipina [Brain aging and calcium antagonist drugs. A preliminary open study with nimodipine]. Clin Ter (Italy) 140(1): 11-15, Jan 1992.

De Marino V, Pisanti N and Capone D. Effects of nimodipine on psychological-stress situation in aged rats. Acta Neurol (Napoli) (Italy) 13(5): 410-7, Oct 1991.

Deyo RA, Straube KT and Disterhoft JF. Nimodipine facilitates associative learning in aging rabbits. Science 243(4892): 809-11, 10 February 1989.

Discover magazine. Rabbit punch [drug enables old rabbits to learn as well as young rabbits]. 10: p12, June 1989.

Grobe-Einsler R and Traber J. Clinical results with nimodipine in Alzheimer disease. Clin Neuropharmacol (United States) 15(suppl 1, Pt A): 416A-17A, 1992.

Hoffmeister F, Benz U, Heise A, et al.. Behavioral effects of nimodipine in animals. Arzneim-Forsch 32: 347-60, 1982.

Hoffmeister F, Benz U, Heise A, et al.. Behavioral effects of nimodipine in animals. Arzneim-Forsch 32: 347-60, 1982.

Isaacson RL, Johnston JE and Vargas DM. The effect of a calcium antagonist on the retention of simple associational learning. Physiol Behav 42(5): 447-52, 1988.

Itil TM, Michael ST, Hoffmeister F, et al.. Nimodipine, a calcium antagonist vasodilator with psychotropic properties (a controlled quantitative pharmaco-EEG study). Curr Ther Res 35: 405-22, 1984.

Itil TM and Itil KZ. The comparative CNS pharmacology of nimodipine in humans. In: Betz E, Deck K, Hoffmeister F, (Eds.) *Nimodipine: pharmacological and clinical properties*. pp. 185-202, Stuttgart: Schattauer Verlag; 1985:

Langley MS and Sorkin EM. Nimodipine: a review of its pharmacodynamic and pharmacokinetic properties, and therapeutic potential in cerebrovascular disease. *Drugs* 37: 669-99, 1989.

Levere TE and Walker A. Old age and cognition: enhancement of recent memory in aged rats by the calcium channel blocker nimodipine. *Neurobiol Aging* (United States) 13(1): 63-6, Jan-Feb 1992.

Levy A, Kong RM, Stillman MJ, Shukitt-Hale B, Kadar T, Rauch TM, Lieberman HR. Nimodipine improves spatial working memory and elevates hippocampal acetylcholine in young rats. *Pharmacol Biochem Behav* (United States) 39(3): 781-6, Jul 1991.

Little HJ, Dolin SJ and Halsey MJ. Calcium channel antagonists decrease the ethanol withdrawal syndrome. *Life Sci* 39: 2059-65, 1986.

Meyer FB, Anderson RE, Sundt TM Jr, *et al.*. Selective central nervous system calcium channel blockers — a new class of anticonvulsant agents. *Mayo Clin Proc* 61: 239-47, 1986.

Morocutti C, Pierelli F, Sanarelli L, *et al.*. Antiepileptic effects of a calcium antagonist (nimodipine) on cefazolin-induced epileptogenic foci in rabbits. *Epilepsia* 27: 498-503, 1986.

Sandin M, Jasmin S and Levere TE. Aging and cognition: facilitation of recent memory in aged nonhuman primates by nimodipine. *Neurobiol Aging* 11(5): 573-5, Sep-Oct 1990.

Schinco P. Mid-term treatment of dementia with nimodipine. *Arch Gerontol Geriatr* (Netherlands) 12(suppl 2): 169-72, 1991.

Schmage N and Bergener M. Global rating, symptoms, behavior, and cognitive performance as indicators of efficacy in clinical studies with nimodipine in elderly patients with cognitive impairment syndromes. *Int Psychogeriatr* (United States) 4(suppl.1): 89-99, 1992.

Scriabine A, Schuurman T and Traber J. Pharmacological basis for the use of nimodipine in central nervous system disorders. *FASEB J* 3(7): 1799-806, May 1989.

Straube KT, Deyo RA, Moyer JR Jr and Disterhoft JF. Dietary nimodipine improves associative learning in aging rabbits. *Neurobiol Aging* 11(6): 659-61, Nov-Dec 1990.

Tollefson GD. Short-term effects of the calcium channel blocker nimodipine (Bay-e-9736) in the management of primary degenerative dementia. *Biol Psychiatry* 27(10): 1133-42, 15 May 1990.

Xu WX and Guo YP. A clinical study of recovery of memories in 46 cases of cerebrovascular diseases [English summary]. *Chung Hua Nei Ko Tsa Chih* (China) 30(12): 752-4, December 1991.

Nimodipine

Phosphatidylserine

Phosphatidylserine is a phospholipid component of brain cell membranes. It acts as a biological detergent, keeping fatty substances soluble and keeping cell membranes fluid. It also seems to augment brain glucose metabolism and increase neurotransmitter receptor sites. Phosphatidylserine has been well studied as a cognitive enhancer in both animals and humans. We found 3569 records on phosphatidylserine in a computer search of Medline. Many of those studies were concerned with memory in humans.

Phosphatidylserine seems to work by increasing glucose metabolism in the brain, and by increasing the number of neurotransmitter receptor sites in the brain [Klinkhammer, *et al.*, 1990]. The increased number of receptor sites may explain why the memory-enhancing effects of phosphatidylserine last for as long as a month after the drug is last taken. In this chapter, we will review a few of the studies done with humans.

Phosphatidylserine is chemically related to other phospholipids such as: phosphatidylcholine, phosphatidylethanolamine and phosphatidylinositol (see illustration, next page). These phospholipids play a vital role as structural components of cell membranes and as biological detergents.

Phosphatidylserine For Normal, Healthy Humans

Thomas Crook and his colleagues did a study on 149 individuals who met their criteria for age-associated memory impairment (AAMI). These people had no overt illnesses, but showed signs of the memory loss that normally occurs with aging. Each individual was given either phosphatidylserine (100 mg three times daily), or a placebo for 12 weeks. Those who took the phosphatidylserine improved on a series of tests designed to measure performance related to learning and memory tasks of

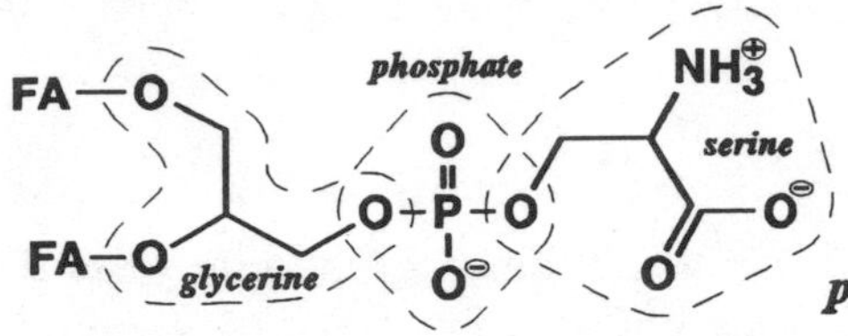

phosphatidylserine

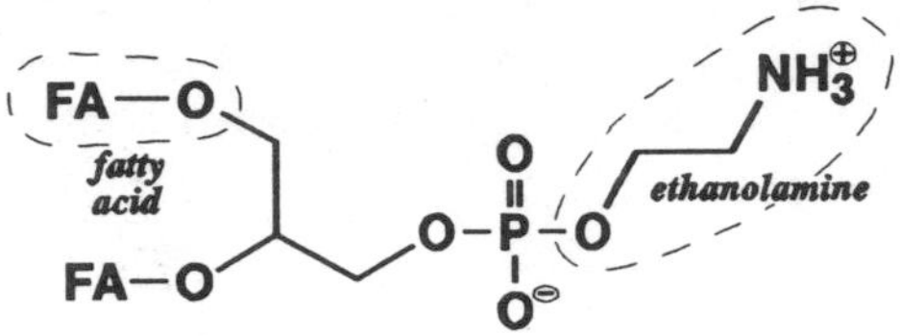

phosphatidyl
ethanolamine

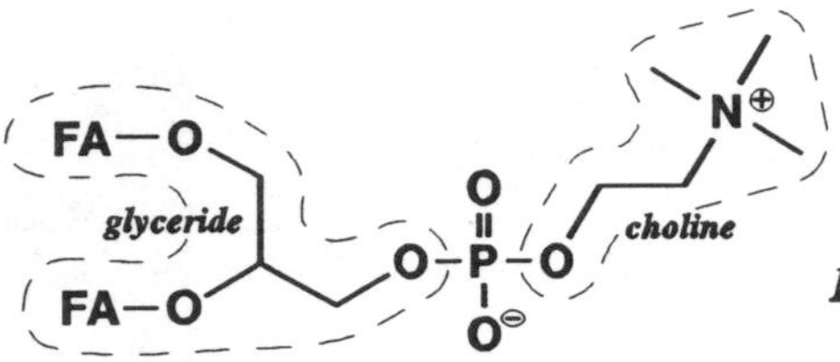

phosphatidylcholine

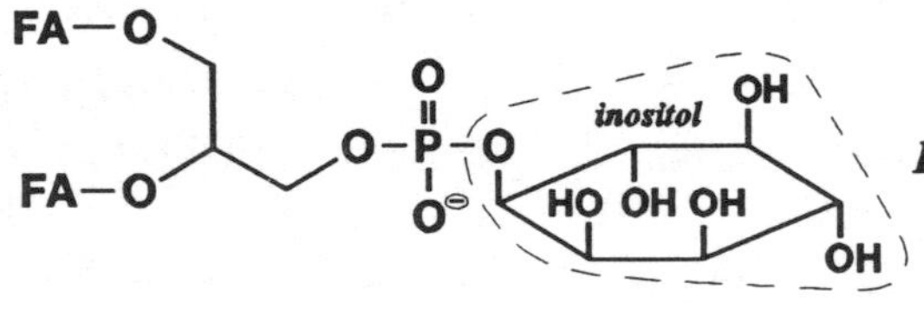

phosphatidyl
inositol

daily life. As in many other smart-drug studies, the people who functioned the worst to begin with were the ones most likely to improve. The researchers concluded that "the compound may be a promising candidate for treating memory loss in later life." [Crook, *et al.*, 1991].

Phosphatidylserine for Depression in the Elderly

It appears that phosphatidylserine may also be effective in treating depression in the elderly. In a study at the University of Milan, in Italy, 10 elderly women with depressive disorders were treated with placebo for 15 days. They were then given phosphatidylserine (300 mg/day) for 30 days. Four different tests were administered before the study began, after the course of placebo, and then again after the 30 day treatment with phosphatidylserine. Phosphatidylserine alleviated depression, and improved memory and general behavior. No adverse effects were noted in any of the patients [Maggioni, *et al.*, 1990].

In another study, researchers administered 400 mg per day of phosphatidylserine for 60 days to 30 elderly outpatients. Psychological tests showed that they experienced profound alleviation of depression. The *dexamethasone suppression test* (a test which psychiatrists use as to diagnose depression) was also normalized by phosphatidylserine in these subjects. Phosphatidylserine not only caused improvements in most of the patients, but the improvements persisted long after phosphatidylserine was discontinued [Rabboni, *et al.*, 1990].

Phosphatidylserine for Alzheimer's Disease

A 1992 study at the University of Munich demonstrated that phosphatidylserine was an effective therapy for patients with early Alzheimer's disease. The study was conducted on 33 patients, and was done in a double-blind cross-over design. Global Improvement Ratings and EEG readings both improved significantly. However, some measures of dementia (GBS dementia-rating scale, psychometric tests, and P300 latency) did not improve [Engel, *et al.*, 1992].

In the U.S., another study tested phosphatidylserine on 51 Alzheimer's patients. Improvements in cognitive performance were most apparent among patients who entered the study with the least cognitive impairment [Crook, *et al.*, 1992].

How Does Phosphatidylserine Compare with Other Smart Drugs?

One Italian study indicates that deprenyl may be even better than phosphatidylserine in cases of mild to moderate Alzheimer's disease (see the Deprenyl and Suggested Treatment Protocol for Alzheimer's Disease chapters for details).   Forty patients with mild-to-moderate Alzheimer's dementia were tested in a randomized, single-blind, parallel fashion. Deprenyl was administered to one group in 10 mg tablets once daily, and phosphatidylserine was given to another group in 100 mg capsules twice daily. Both treatment regimens went on for three months. At the beginning of the study, and then each month thereafter during the study, the patients were given an extensive battery of neuropsychological tests. The deprenyl group showed greater improvements than the phosphatidylserine group on most of the tests. In addition, the deprenyl group showed an increased degree of autonomy in day-to-day activities. This effect was not found in the phosphatidylserine group, however. The only adverse side effects reported in either group were rare cases of mild nausea [Monteverde, *et al.*, 1990].

Many other studies have clearly shown that phosphatidylserine is effective for treatment of senility, Alzheimer's, AAMI, depression, and for cognition enhancement in normal, healthy humans. Phosphatidylserine may even be useful in the regulation of immune function [Scapagnini, *et al.*, 1990; Sinforiani, *et al.*, 1987; Caffarra, *et al.*, 1987; Wilkerson, 1992; Rosadini, *et al.*, 1990, 1991; Rabboni, *et al.*, 1990; Granata, *et al.*, 1987; Puca, *et al.*, 1987; Villardita, *et al.*, 1987; Palmieri, *et al.*, 1987; Ransmayr, *et al.*, 1987; Delwaide, *et al.*, 1986].

Precautions

Phosphatidylserine may interact negatively with anticoagulants. Occasional mild nausea is the only other reported side effect.

Dosage

100-200 mg twice daily orally, or 100-250 mg daily by IM (intramuscular) or slow IV (intravenous) injection. When combining smart drugs you may need to reduce the dosages.

Sources

Phosphatidylserine is manufactured by the Italian pharmaceutical company Fidia. For an up-to-date product sources list you can send in the tearout card at the front of this book. See also Appendix A.

References

Amaducci L. Phosphatidylserine in the treatment of Alzheimer's disease: results of a multicenter study. *Psychopharmacol Bull* 24(1): 130-4, 1988.

Amaducci L, Crook TH, Lippi A, Bracco L, Baldereschi M, Latorraca S, Piersanti P, Tesco G and Sorbi S. Use of phosphatidylserine in Alzheimer's disease. *Ann N Y Acad Sci* (United States) 640: 245-9, 1991.

Caffarra P and Santamaria V. The effects of phosphatidylserine in patients with mild cognitive decline. An open trial. *Clin Trials J* (United Kingdom) 24(1): 109-14, 1987.

Crook T, Petrie W, Wells C and Massari DC. Effects of phosphatidylserine in Alzheimer's disease. *Psychopharmacol Bull* (United States) 28(1): 61-6, 1992.

Crook TH, Tinklenberg J, Yesavage J, Petrie W, Nunzi MG and Massari DC. Effects of phosphatidylserine in age-associated memory impairment. *Neurology* 41(5): 644-9, May 1991.

Delwaide PJ, Gyselynck-Mambourg AM, Hurlet A and Ylieff M. Double-blind randomized controlled study of phosphatidylserine in senile demented patients. *Acta Neurol Scand* (Denmark) 73(2): 136-40, February 1986.

Engel RR, Satzger W, Gunther W, Kathmann N, Bove D, Gerke S, Munch U and Hippius H. Double-blind cross-over study of phosphatidylserine vs. placebo in patients with early dementia of the Alzheimer type. *Eur Neuropsychopharmacol* (Netherlands) 2(2): 149-55, Jun 1992.

Granata Q and Di Michele J. Phosphatidylserine in elderly patients. An open trial. *Clin Trials J* (United Kingdom) 24(1): 99-103, 1987.

Klinkhammer P, Szelies B and Heiss WD. Effect of phosphatidylserine on cerebral glucose metabolism in Alzheimer's disease. *Dementia* (Switzerland) 1(4): 197-201, 1990.

Maggioni M, Picotti GB, Bondiolotti GP, Panerai A, Cenacchi T, Nobile P and Brambilla F. Effects of phosphatidylserine therapy in geriatric patients with depressive disorders. *Acta Psychiatr Scand* 81(3): 265-70, March 1990.

Marcon GM and Mascolo MD. Esperienza su un trattamento con fosfatidilserina in pazienti con declino cognitivo e del comportamento [Experience with phosphatidylserine treatment of patients with cognitive and behavioral decline]. *Clin Ter* 126(4): 243-8, 31 Aug 1988.

Monteverde A, Gnemmi P, Rossi F, Monteverde A and Finali GC. Selegiline in the treatment of mild to moderate Alzheimer-type dementia. *Clin Ther* 12(4): 315-22, Jul-Aug 1990.

Palmieri G, Palmieri R, Inzoli MR, *et al.*. Double-blind controlled trial of phosphatidylserine in patients with senile mental deterioration. *Clin Trials J* (United Kingdom) 24(1): 73-83, 1987.

Phosphatidylserine

Puca FM, Savarese MA and Minervini MG. Exploratory trial of phosphatidylserine efficacy in mildly demented patients. *Clin Trials J* (United Kingdom) 24(1): 94-98, 1987.

Rabboni M, Maggioni FS, Giannelli A and Beinat L. Neuroendocrine and behavioural effects of phosphatidylserine in elderly patients with abiotrophic or vascular dementia or mild depression. A preliminary trial. *Clin Trials J* (United Kingdom) 27(3): 230-40, 1990.

Ransmayr G, Plorer S, Gerstenbrand F and Bauer G. Double-blind placebo-controlled trial of phosphatidylserine in elderly patients with arteriosclerotic encephalopathy. *Clin Trials J* (United Kingdom) 24(1): 62-72, 1987.

Rosadini G, Sannita WG, Nobili F and Cenacchi T. Phosphatidylserine: Quantitative EEG effects in healthy volunteers. *Neuropsychobiology* (Switzerland) 24(1): 42-8, 1990.

Scapagnini U, Guarcello V, Triolo G, Cioni M, Morale MC, Farinella Z and Marchetti B. Therapeutic perspectives in psychoneuroendocrinimmunology (PNEI): potential role of phosphatidylserine in neuroendocrine-immune communications. *Int J Neurosci* 51(3-4): 299-301, April 1990.

Sinforiani E, Agostinis C, Merlo P, *et al.*. Cognitive decline in aging brain. Therapeutic approach with phosphatidylserine. *Clin Trials J* (United Kingdom) 24(1): 115-24, 1987.

The SMID Group. Phosphatidylserine in the treatment of clinically diagnosed Alzheimer's disease. *J Neural Transm* Suppl 24: 287-92, 1987.

Villardita C, Grioli S, Salmeri G, *et al.*. Multicentre clinical trial of brain phosphatidyl-serine in elderly patients with intellectual deterioration. *Clin Trials J* (United Kingdom) 24(1): 84-93, 1987.

Wilkerson WW. Agents for the treatment of Alzheimer's disease: Recent patent advances July to December 1991. *Curr Opin Ther Pat* (United Kingdom) 2(2): 135-45, 1992.

Pregnenolone

Pregnenolone is a steroid-hormone precursor. It is manufactured from cholesterol in the body and undergoes conversion into a host of steroid chemicals including DHEA, estrogen, testosterone and progesterone (see the following illustration). What makes pregnenolone unique among these steroids is its unusual memory-enhancing activity. In a recent rat study [Flood, 1991], it was found to be 100 times more effective at improving memory and learning tasks than other steroids. Pregnenolone is also unique among the smart drugs presented in this book for the lack of human research documenting this memory-enhancing effect.

Steroids and Aging

Pregnenolone, and other steroid precursor hormones like DHEA (dehydroepiandrosterone) (see the following illustration) undergo a strong age-related decrease in concentration. DHEA (a metabolite of pregnenolone) has been shown to ameliorate many age-related symptoms in both animal and human studies, and it also has dramatically extended lifespan in rodents. It is under close scrutiny as an anti-obesity treatment in women and for its anti-cancer influences. Although pregnenolone and DHEA are steroids, they do *not* exhibit the strong hormone influences of fully formed steroids like estrogen (estradiol), testosterone, or progesterone. As a consequence, steroid precursors like pregnenolone and DHEA possess minimal anabolic, androgenic and estrogenic activity.

Despite the lack of human experience with pregnenolone as a smart drug, it is well known historically as a treatment for arthritis. Used extensively in the 1940s, pregnenolone has since fallen into disuse with the advent of newer, high-tech, anti-inflammatory steroid drugs. Pregnenolone's multiple-decade record of safety and its low toxicity will enable relatively quick

investigation of its memory effects in humans. We expect preliminary results in the next year.

Pregnenolone and Memory

In 1992, Drs. Flood, Morley, and Roberts published the results
of their ground-breaking study. In the study, experimental mice
were placed in a T-shaped maze and given 5 seconds after a bell
sounded to find their way into the correct arm of the T. If they
failed to do so within 5 seconds, they were electrically shocked
until they succeeded. Once trained in the "foot-shock active-
avoidance" procedure, the mice were injected with a steroid
hormone or a placebo. One week later, they were retested for
retention of the learned response.

Almost all steroids were found to reduce the number of runs
required for the mice to relearn the shock-avoidance procedure
(*i.e.*, to successfully run the T-maze 5 out of 6 *consecutive*
attempts). Pregnenolone was unique in being active at doses
one hundred times lower than any other steroid compound.

Most hormones were found to exhibit an "inverted-U-shaped
dose-response curve" which covered a two- to five-fold dose
range. DHEA, however, was effective at decreasing the
number of runs at doses over a hundred-fold range, and
pregnenolone, at an up-to-ten-thousand-fold dose range. See
the How To Use Smart Drugs chapter in *Smart Drugs &
Nutrients* for more details about inverted-U-shaped dose-
response curves.

The scientists were unable to identify any relationship between
the presence or absence of memory-enhancing activity and the
structural features of the different steroids. They were also
unable to identify any particular influence on neuroreceptor
systems. At the present time, the mechanism by which steroids
influence memory and learning remains elusive.

Although pregnenolone is completely non-toxic and cheap,
human trials of its memory-enhancing properties are only now
taking place. Exactly how shock-avoidance improvements in

Cholesterol → *Pregnenolone* → Progesterone

17α-Hydroxypregnenolone → 17α-Hydroxyprogesterone

DHEA
Dehydroepiandrosterone ⇌ Androstenedione → Estrone

Androstenediol → Testosterone → Estradiol

Dihydrotestosterone

Steroid Biosynthesis Pathways

mice may translate into cognitive enhancement in humans remains to be seen.

Dr. Bruce Miller, neurologist at the Harbor-UCLA Medical Center in Torrance, California, is currently examining pregnenolone's effect on patients with mild-to-severe Alzheimer's disease, as well as healthy older people with age-related memory impairment.

Dosage

Ideal pregnenolone and DHEA dosages can vary dramatically from person to person. Age is a strong factor, but other biological influences may be significant. DHEA dosages range from 25-500 mg and pregnenolone from 5-100 mg. When combining smart drugs you may need to reduce the dosages.

Precautions

Before-and-after tests of blood DHEA and DHEA-sulfate levels are recommended to assess the dose of either steroid. Medical supervision is suggested.

Sources

Pregnenolone may be available through some pharmacies with a doctor's prescription; however, it has not been in common use for many years, and so may be difficult to find. We know of two compounding pharmacies offering pregnenolone and DHEA as available ingredients (see Appendix A for product sources information). Some overseas smart-drug suppliers may have these items in inventory, however, there are rumors that the DEA may classify steroid precursors as controlled substances in an attempt to prevent anabolic steroids from being manufactured for bodybuilders. For an up-to-date product sources list from CERI, send in the tearout card at the front of this book.

References

Flood JF, Morley JE and Roberts E. Memory-enhancing effects in male mice of pregnenolone and steroids metabolically derived from it. *Proc Natl Acad Sci* 89: 1567-71, March 1992.

Ondansetron and Zatosetron

Neurotransmitters work by interacting with "sensing stations" known as *receptors* which are on the nerve cell outer membrane surfaces. These receptors can be stimulated or inhibited only by certain specific substances which have affinity for the receptor site. One group of receptors are the *5-HT receptors*, which are specific for the inhibitory neurotransmitter *serotonin* (5-hydroxytryptamine, or 5-HT for short). A number of sub-types of this receptor system have been identified, all of which cause slight differences in actions when stimulated or inhibited [Tyers, 1992]. One sub-type of 5-HT receptors, the 5-HT_3 receptors, are found on cholinergic neurons. When these receptors are activated by serotonin, they inhibit the release of acetylcholine from these neurons. *Ondansetron*, a new drug developed by Glaxo Pharmaceuticals, blocks these receptors, thereby *increasing* the release of acetylcholine from these neurons. Acetylcholine deficits are a common aspect of most forms of memory impairment.

Changes in serotonin are believed to occur with advancing age. Research with 5-HT_3 antagonists (like ondansetron) indicates that these types of drugs may improve memory in some healthy older adults with age-associated memory impairment (AAMI). Crook and colleagues [1991] measured the effects of ondansetron on multiple measures of AAMI. The results with immediate and delayed "name-face recall" indicate that improvements in memory still accrue after 12 weeks of ondansetron administration (see figure).

According to a Glaxo corporate video, "5-HT_3 receptors control a wide variety of functions. One example is *memory*. As we get older, our brain becomes less efficient at storing information, and we may become a little absent-minded. This is to be expected. But in some people, it happens prematurely — with debilitating effects."

Effect of Ondansetron and Placebo on Immediate & Delayed Name–Face Recall

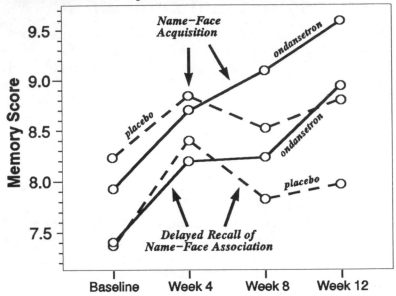

According to Dr. Paul Williams, the director of CNS clinical research at Glaxo, "We studied between 200 and 250 patients with age-associated memory impairment. We found that 12 week's treatment with ondansetron (Zofran) significantly improved the patient's memories, as compared to placebo. The extent of the improvement in memory functioning was roughly equivalent to the amount of memory that is lost every six years with aging. We are extremely excited by these results [*Horizon*, 1991]."

Although the drug is approved by the FDA only for use as an anti-emetic (anti-vomiting and anti-nausea) drug for use following cancer chemotherapy, the British drug company is clearly targeting the huge potential market of people with AAMI.

Through behavioral testing, Glaxo researchers have been able to show that ondansetron, by selectively blocking serotonin, actually increases acetylcholine release and enhances memory and performance. Dr. Mike Tyers, Central Nervous System Research Director at Glaxo, stated:

> *"The great advantage that [ondansetron] will have over other approaches...is that it will only increase acetylcholine in that part of the brain which is concerned with memory. In this sense, ondansetron could improve cognitive function without actually causing the side effects associated with acetylcholine release in other parts of the body [Horizon, 1991]."*

What Was That About Memory?

Several studies since 1990 have demonstrated that ondansetron improves memory and learning ability in mice, rats, marmosets, and primates. In some of these studies, researchers first administered scopolamine to the animals, to cause memory deficits. Ondansetron was then used successfully to reverse the "scopalamine-induced cognitive deficit." Other studies have shown that ondansetron enhances cognition in normal, healthy animals [Carey, *et al.*, 1992; Domeney, *et al.*, 1991; Barnes, *et al.*, 1990].

Ongoing Research with a New 5-HT$_3$ Antagonist

Although ondansetron is available by prescription in the U.S., it is currently available only in an IV injectable form. Zatosetron is another serotonin antagonist that is available in pill form in England. Although zatosetron is very new, its potential for improving cognition in older adults with age-associated memory impairment has not escaped researchers. It is currently under investigation at Memory Assessment Clinics, Inc. (MAC) at their facilities in Bethesda, Maryland, and Scottsdale, Arizona. MAC is conducting a preliminary double-blind study of 200 patients over the age of 50 years who have experienced changes in memory associated with the normal aging process (*i.e.*, AAMI). Dosages will range from 0.2 to 20 mg of zatosetron per day in the treatment group. Another group will receive a placebo.

MAC scientists are still recruiting clients for the study. To determine your eligibility to participate in this project, contact Memory Assessment Clinics, Inc., 8311 Wisconsin Avenue, Suite A-6, Bethesda, MD, 20814, Phone: (301) 657-0030.

Other Uses of Ondansetron

Anti-nausea and memory enhancement are not the only potential uses for ondansetron. It is also being investigated as a treatment for schizophrenia, anxiety, alcohol abuse, and drug withdrawal [Costall, *et al.*, 1992].

Ondansetron is a powerful anti-anxiety drug, which can be used instead of benzodiazepine drugs like Valium. Unlike Valium, however, it has no sedative effect, no potential for addiction, and no withdrawal symptoms when the drug is discontinued. In fact, a remarkable feature of ondansetron and other serotonin antagonist-class drugs (including $5-HT_1$ antagonists *buspirone* [Buspar], Gepirone, and Ipsapirone), is that they do not seem to alter normal behavior [Broocks, 1992; Sellers, *et al.*, 1992; Cowen, 1991]. My experience with these drugs [WD] confirms that they make formerly anxious people feel "normal."

Precautions

Ondansetron has been known to occasionally cause gastro-intestinal disturbance or rash. Rare cases of bronchospasm, tachycardia, angina (chest pain), hypokalemia, electrocardio-graphic alterations, and seizures have been reported but it was not clear if these were caused by the ondansetron.

Dosage

The recommended IV dosage of ondansetron is three 0.15 mg/kg doses per day. Please see the *Physician's Desk Reference* for more information on IV use. Oral forms may be available in other countries (and obtainable by mail-order from those countries). Please see the dosage instructions in the drug insert for these products. Also remember: when combining smart drugs you may need to reduce the dosages.

Sources

Oral forms of ondansetron are not yet available in the United States but may become available from some overseas mail-order sources. Please send in the tearout card at the front of this book to get an up-to-date product sources list.

References

Barnes JM, Costall B, Coughlan J, Domeney AM, Gerrard PA, Kelly ME, Naylor RJ, Onaivi ES, Tomkins DM and Tyers MB. The effects of ondansetron, a 5-HT3 receptor antagonist, on cognition in rodents and primates. *Pharmacol Biochem Behav* 35(4): 955-62, April 1990.

Broocks A. Ondansetron — Der erste hochselektive 5-HT3-antagonist in der therapie psychiatrischer erkrankungen [Ondansetron — The first highly selective 5-HT3 antagonist in the treatment of mental diseases. *Fortschr Neurol Psychiatr* (Germany) , 1992, 60(6): 227-36, 1992.

Carey GJ, Costall B, Domeney AM, Gerrard PA, Jones DN, Naylor RJ and Tyers MB. Ondansetron and arecoline prevent scopolamine-induced cognitive deficits in the marmoset. *Pharmacol Biochem Behav.* 1992, 42 (1) p75-83

Costall B and Naylor RJ. Serotonin and psychiatric disorders. A key to new therapeutic approaches. *Arzneimittelforschung* 42(2A): 246-9, 1992.

Costall B and Naylor RJ. The psychopharmacology of 5-HT3 receptors. *Pharmacol Toxicol* (Denmark) 71(6): 401-15, 1992.

Cowen PJ. Serotonin receptor subtypes: Implications for psychopharmacology. *Br J Psychiatry* (United Kingdom) 159(suppl 12): 7-14, September 1991.

Crook T and Lakin M. Effects of ondansetron in age-associated memory impairment. *Biol Psychiatry* 2: 888-90, 1991.

Domeney AM, Costall B, Gerrard PA, Jones DN, Naylor RJ and Tyers MB. The effect of ondansetron on cognitive performance in the marmoset. *Pharmacol Biochem Behav* 38(1): 169-75, January 1991.

Horizon. BBC Production, 1991.

Ondansetron Gegen Gedachtnisschwache [Ondansetron in the treatment of memory disturbances]. *Dtsch Apoth Ztg* (Germany) 131(26): 1365, 1991.

Peroutka SJ, Sleight AJ, McCarthy BG, Pierce PA, Schmidt AW and Hekmatpanah CR. The clinical utility of pharmacological agents that act at serotonin receptors. *J Neuropsychiatry* 1(3): 253-62, 1989.

Sellers EM, Higgins GA and Sobell MB. 5-HT and alcohol abuse. *Trends Pharmacol Sci.* (United Kingdom) 13(2): 69-75, 1992.

Tyers MB. Pharmacology and preclinical antiemetic properties of ondansetron. *Seminars in Oncology* 19(4): (suppl. 10), 1-8, 1992.

Ondansetron and Zatosetron

Acetyl-L-Carnitine Update

Acetyl-L-carnitine (ALC) was one of the most exciting substances covered in *Smart Drugs & Nutrients*. ALC now looks even *more* promising as a cognition enhancer for normal, healthy people, and as a treatment for age-associated memory impairment (AAMI) and Alzheimer's disease. Many human trials have been done with ALC since publication of *Smart Drugs & Nutrients*. We found 52 human trials done with ALC since 1990 alone!

Acetyl-L-carnitine has been available in Italy since 1986, where it is classified as a nootropic drug and is used to treat Alzheimer's disease and AAMI. ALC occurs naturally in the body, where it transports fats into mitochondria (mitochondria are the powerhouses of the cells). ALC is also found in common foods like milk.

ALC is closely related to *carnitine*, a naturally occurring amino acid (ALC is an O-acetyl derivative of carnitine). Carnitine has been used in the fields of myocardial ischemia and skeletal muscle pathology. Scientists noted that elderly heart patients treated with carnitine demonstrated improved mood and increased affective tone. This led to many studies of the effects of ALC on cognitive disorders.

ALC Improves Performance in Normal Healthy Humans

There have been many studies showing that ALC improves learning and memory in normal, healthy mice and rats [Bossoni, 1986, Drago, 1986; Ghirardi, *et al.*, 1992; Barnes, *et al.*, 1990]. Until recently, most of the studies in humans have been performed on patients with Alzheimer's disease or AAMI.

However, in June, 1992, Italian researchers published a landmark study which confirmed that ALC improves performance in young, healthy people. The researchers chose 17 healthy subjects (8 males and 9 females) between 22 and 27 years old. Ten of the subjects were physically active, and played competitive sports regularly, while 7 were sedentary and didn't exercise. Each subject was given either 1500 mg of ALC per day or placebo for 30 days. Each person in the study was tested before and after treatment using a videogame-type device designed to evaluate attention levels and hand-eye coordination and reflexes. Reflex speed was markedly increased in those using ALC. Also, the number of errors and the task completion time was reduced in those who took ALC by 3 to 4 times over controls. There were no adverse effects in *any* of the subjects. This study indicates that ALC can improve performance in normal, healthy people [Lino, *et al.*, 1992].

Researchers believe that ALC improves cognition by enhancing the activity of acetylcholine and/or increasing neuronal metabolism. It may also work by increasing dopamine activity in the part of the brain where dopamine is made [Harsing, *et al.*, 1992; Sershen, *et al.*, 1991].

ALC for Treatment of AAMI

In 1989, 20 patients were treated with 1500 mg ALC per day for six months. All patients had *involutional symptoms*, the regressive mental and physical changes which sometimes occur with old age. They were being treated by a rehabilitation therapist for their decreased physical abilities. After treatment with ALC, all patients demonstrated improved cognitive ability, less depression, greater self-sufficiency, improved social life and increased motor activity [Fiore, 1989].

The following year, two other Italian researchers evaluated 236 mentally-impaired elderly people being treated with ALC in a large multicenter study. Each subject was treated for over five months with 1500 mg of ALC per day or a placebo. All participants were given tests for cognitive function, emotional state, and social behavior. Those who took ALC improved significantly on all measures tested. Significant improvement was noted especially for memory, constructional thinking, and emotional state [Cipolli and Chiari, 1990].

Most recently, researchers at the University of Modena in Italy found that ALC not only improved cognitive performance in elderly subjects, but also that *the cognitive gains persisted long after the treatment ended*. This study was single-blind (meaning that the researchers, but not the patients, knew who was using ALC and who was using a placebo), and was carried out on 279 subjects from 42 centers. Testing was done for cognitive function, emotional state, and relational behavior. Thirty days after completion of the ALC treatment, the tests were repeated. The ALC recipients demonstrated that they had retained significant gains on all measures as compared to the placebo group [Vecchi, *et al.*, 1991].

ALC Counteracts Depression in the Elderly

Depression is one of the most common disorders to cause people to seek medical treatment. In Italy, researchers studied the effects of ALC in patients with depression. Sixty depressed people between the ages of 60 and 80 were given either 3000 mg ALC or a placebo for 60 days. They were tested before treatment began and then repeatedly throughout the study. These tests — which evaluated depression and general well-being — showed that ALC reduced the severity of depression and improved the quality of life [Bella, *et al.*, 1990].

Another placebo-controlled study of 28 patients between 70 and 80 years old also showed that ALC alleviated symptoms of depression. Each participant was given either 1500 mg of ALC per day or a placebo. The ALC-treated group showed improvement on two separate psychiatric depression scales (the Hamilton Rating Scale for Depression, and the Beck Depression Inventory). They also showed subjectively beneficial changes in behavior [Garzya, *et al.*, 1990].

Sleep disturbances and other disruptions of circadian rhythm are a hallmark of clinical depression. These circadian disturbances can have a profoundly adverse effect on memory (see the Melatonin chapter). Three Italian scientists found that ALC alleviated depression and also normalized daily cortisol rhythms in their depressed patients [Gecele, *et al.*, 1991].

ALC also appears to reduce sleep requirements while improving the quality of sleep. These results were confirmed in 8 out of 10 subjects with cerebrovascular disease [Scrofani, *et al.*, 1988]. Similar results have been obtained in people with senile depression in doses ranging from 500 mg to 3000 mg per day [Fulgente, *et al.*, 1990; Garzya, *et al.*, 1990; Villardita, *et al.*, 1984; Tempesta, *et al.*, 1987].

ALC for Treatment of Alzheimer's Disease

ALC is now regarded by scientists and pharmaceutical companies as one of the most promising drugs for treatment of Alzheimer's disease. In November 1991, Hoffmann-La Roche completed negotiations with Sigma-Tau (the Italian developer of acetyl-L-carnitine) for worldwide marketing rights to ALC. One chemical news journal indicated that Sigma-Tau expected a turnover of $600 million in 1991 alone [Chim. Actual., 1991].

At Columbia University in New York, researchers conducted a double-blind, parallel-design, placebo-controlled study of ALC in 30 patients with early Alzheimer's disease. Each individual was given tests of memory, attention, language, and visuospatial and constructional abilities. Levels of ALC in cerebrospinal fluid were also measured (this test requires a spinal tap — ouch!). Then, each patient was given ALC or a placebo. After six months, the group which received ALC showed less deterioration in several of the above tests. The authors concluded that "ALC may retard the deterioration in some cognitive areas in patients with Alzheimer's disease." The dosages used in this study were 2.5 to three grams/day for three months [Sano, *et al.*, 1992].

At the Georgia State University Department of Nutrition and Dietetics, another study was conducted in which people with Alzheimer's disease were given 2000 mg of ALC per day for a full year. This double-blind, randomized, controlled clinical trial showed that the progression of the disease was significantly reduced in patients receiving the ALC instead of the placebo [Bowman, 1992].

In England, six scientists at Whittington Hospital conducted an experiment which showed that ALC is safe and partially effective in people with full-blown Alzheimer's disease. A total of 36 patients were enrolled and were given either 2000 mg of ALC per day or placebo. The researchers concluded that ALC "may have a beneficial effect on some clinical features of Alzheimer-type dementia, particularly those related to short-term memory" [Rai, 1990]. The only side effect noted was nausea in a few of the patients, particularly when the drug was taken on an empty stomach.

Several other studies have confirmed that ALC improves memory, attention span, and alertness in people with Alzheimer's disease [Cabrero, *et al.*, 1992; Cazzato, *et al.*, 1990].

Because of its effectiveness and overwhelming safety record, we believe ALC should be always be considered for the treatment of Alzheimer's disease.

ALC Compared to Deprenyl

In 1990, Italian researchers compared ALC with deprenyl for treatment of Alzheimer's dementia. Forty people with mild-to-moderate Alzheimer's disease (13 men and 27 women aged 56 to 80) participated in this single-blind, randomized, parallel study. For 90 days, patients were given either deprenyl (10 mg per day) or ALC (500 mg twice per day). Extensive testing was done at the beginning of the study and every 30 days thereafter. Deprenyl improved patients' abilities to process, store, and retrieve information. Improvements in verbal fluency and visuospatial abilities were also noted. At these dosages, deprenyl was far more effective than ALC with respect to the degree of improvement. No adverse reactions occurred in either group [Campi, *et al.*, 1990].

The study just described may be flawed, however, because of the relatively low dose of ALC that was used. Many of the studies we discussed above used 2000 mg or even 3000 mg of ALC per day. This study used only 1000 mg. The dose of deprenyl, on the other hand, was fairly high — 10 mg per day. Nevertheless, this report is interesting in that it showed positive results for both drugs (even at the low doses of ALC used). We wish they had tried both drugs *together*. See the Suggested Treatment Protocol for Alzheimer's Disease chapter.

Senility

In 1986, researchers gave 500 mg of ALC per day to 20 people with senility (20 others were given placebo). Although this study used a fairly low dose, and was short-term (only 40 days), positive effects were found. The researchers concluded that ALC caused a significant improvement in several measures of senility [Bonavita, 1986].

Two years later, a longer, three-month, trial was conducted on 30 people with senility. The researchers administered 2000 mg ALC per day or placebo on a double-blind basis. The ALC-treated group performed better on a variety of tests for memory [Cucinotta, *et al.*, 1988].

In 1990, researchers at the University of Parma in Italy confirmed again that ALC is an effective treatment for mental impairment resulting from senile dementia. The researchers conducted a three-month, double-blind, controlled study with 60 elderly senile patients randomly divided into two groups of 30 each. One group was given 2000 mg of ALC per day, and the other was given placebo. The researchers concluded that the ALC-treated patients "showed statistically significant improvement in the behavioral scales, in the memory tests, in the attention barrage test and in the Verbal Fluency test [Passeri, *et al.*, 1990]."

Other studies of ALC have also shown similar effects for individuals with senile dementia [Sinforiani, *et al.*, 1990; Bonavita, *et al.*, 1988].

ALC for Cerebrovascular Insufficiency

Reduced blood flow to the brain is a common problem in aging because atherosclerosis causes blood vessels to become too narrow to supply the brain with enough blood. ALC improves cerebral blood flow in patients with cerebrovascular disease [Postiglione, *et al.*, 1990; Rosadini, *et al.*, 1988].

In one study, twelve elderly subjects with cerebrovascular insufficiency were given ALC or a placebo. The ALC-treated group showed significant improvement in memory, number and word tests, responses to simple stimuli, and performance on a maze test [Arrigo, *et al.*, 1990]. There were no side effects. An earlier study by the same researchers showed that reaction time also improved [Arrigo, *et al.*, 1988].

ALC for Alcohol-Induced Cognitive Impairment

At the Catholic University of Rome in Italy, 10 researchers looked at the potential of ALC for treating cognitive impairment caused by chronic alcohol abuse. The study used 55 alcoholics who had been abstinent for at least one month. Each person chosen for the study also showed signs of cognitive impairment. In this study, each participant was given either 2000 mg ALC per day or a placebo. Subjects were given a variety of neuropsychological tests at the beginning of the study and then after 45 and 90 days. The ALC group improved on all cognitive areas explored. The researchers concluded that ALC "can be a useful and safe therapeutic agent in the subtle cognitive disturbances of chronic alcoholics" [Tempesta, *et al.*, 1990].

Anti-Aging Effects of ALC

ALC also appears to be able to protect the brain from the effects of aging. NMDA-sensitive glutamate receptors in the brain are important for learning, but decrease in numbers with age. One study of these receptors in rat brains found that ALC has a neuroprotective and neurotrophic (brain-cell nourishing) effect during aging [Fiore, *et al.*,1989].

Long-term administration of ALC preserves spatial memory in aged rats [Ghirardi, 1989], slows down certain age-related cognitive deficits, may slow the aging process itself [Laguzzi, *et al.*, 1992], and may increase lifespan [Markowska, *et al.*, 1990; Caprioli, *et al.*, 1990].

Lipofuscin (aging pigment) is the substance that accumulates on the backs of some older peoples' hands (also called "age" or "liver" spots). Lipofuscin also builds up in heart and nerve cells with aging, and is sometimes associated with a reduction of cognitive powers. ALC actually reduces the formation of lipofuscin in the brains of aged laboratory animals and reduces the lipofuscin levels to those of much younger animals [Kohjimoto, 1988; Amenta, *et al.*, 1989]. Some of my patients have reported that their "age spots" had disappeared after taking ALC for six months [WD].

ALC may also improve immune function. Several immune parameters predictably change for the worse with age. In one study, ALC seemed to restore a number of these immune parameters to the levels of much younger individuals [Franceschi, *et al.*, 1990]. ALC is also being studied for possible benefit in Parkinson's disease [Puca, *et al.*, 1990].

Precautions

The studies reviewed above indicate that ALC is a very safe substance with a wide range of preventive and therapeutic uses. Nevertheless, it is contraindicated in pregnancy, lactation or hypersensitivity to ALC. ALC is a naturally occurring substance found in milk and other common foods. It is also found naturally in the human body.

Dosage

ALC usually comes in 500 mg tablets, or in a liquid solution dispensed by drops. The usual dose is 1000 mg to 2000 mg per day, in two divided doses. When combining smart drugs you may need to reduce the dosages.

Sources

For an up-to-date product sources list you can send in the tearout card at the front of this book.

We know of one nutrient company that is making ALC available (see the listing for Source Naturals in Appendix A.) If you can't obtain ALC, or the FDA pulls ALC off the U.S. over-the-counter market, a closely-related amino acid, carnitine, seems to share many of the metabolic effects of ALC. Carnitine is available over-the-counter in the U.S. as a dietary supplement. Considering the remarkable safety and effectiveness of ALC, we see no reason not to recommend its widespread use. Other names for ALC include: Branigen, Nicetile, Zibren, Alcar, levacecarnine hydrochloride, N-acetyl-L-carnitine, L-acetylcarnitine, and ST-200.

References

Amenta F, Ferrante F, Lucreziotti R, Ricci A and Ramacci MT. Reduced lipofuscin accumulation in senescent rat brain by long-term acetyl-L-carnitine treatment. *Arch Gerontol Geriatr* (Netherlands) 9(2): 147-53, 1989.

Arrigo A, Casale R, Buonocore M and Ciano C. Effects of acetyl-L-carnitine on reaction times in patients with cerebrovascular insufficiency. *Int J Clin Pharmacol Res* 10(1-2): 133-7, 1990.

Arrigo A, Clano E, Casale R and Buonocore M. The effects of L-acetylcarnitine on reaction times in patients with cerebrovascular insufficiency. A double blind cross-over study. *Clin Trials J* (United Kingdom) 25(Suppl. 1): 47-56, 1988.

Barnes CA, Markowska AL, Ingram DK, Kametani H, Spangler EL, Lemken VJ and Olton DS. Acetyl-L-carnitine. 2: Effects on learning and memory performance of aged rats in simple and complex mazes. *Neurobiol Aging* 11(5): 499-506, Sep-Oct 1990.

Bella R, Biondi R, Raffaele R and Pennisi G. Effect of acetyl-L-carnitine on geriatric patients suffering from dysthymic disorders. *Int J Clin Pharmacol Res* 10(6): 355-60, 1990.

Bonavita E. Study of the efficacy and tolerability of L-acetylcarnitine therapy in the senile brain. *Journal of Clinical Pharmacology, Therapy, and Toxicology* 24: 511-6, 1986.

Bonavita E, Bertuzzi D, Bonavita J and Marani A. L-acetylcarnitine (L-Ac) [Branigen] in the long-term symptomatic treatment of senile dementia. Optimal treatment times and suspension periods. *Clin Trials J* (United Kingdom) 25(4): 227-37, 1988.

Bossoni G and Carpi C. Effect of acetyl-L-carnitine on conditioned reflex learning rate and retention in laboratory animals. *Drugs Under Experimental and Clinical Research* 12(11): 911-6, 1986.

Bowman BAB. Acetyl-carnitine and Alzheimer's disease. *Nutrition Review* (USA) 50(5): 142-4, 1992.

Cabrero Lahuerta MC and Cortes Blanco M. Current treatment of Alzheimer's disease [Aproximacion al estado actual del tratamiento de la demencia senil tipo Alzheimer]. *Cienc Med* (Spain) 9(3): 82-7, 1992.

Campi N, Todeschini GP and Scarzella L. Selegiline versus L-acetylcarnitine in the treatment of Alzheimer-type dementia. *Clin Ther* 12(4): 306-14, Jul-Aug 1990.

Caprioli A, Ghirardi O, Ramacci MT and Angelucci L. Age-dependent deficits in radial maze performance in the rat: Effect of chronic treatment with acetyl-L-carnitine. *Prog Neuropsychopharmacol Biol Psychiatry* 14(3): 359-69, 1990.

Cazzato G, Bonfigli L, Pasqua M and Iaiza F. Long-term treatment with acetyl-L-carnitine in patients suffering from dementia of the Alzheimer's type [Trattamento a lungo termine con L-acetilcarnitina in pazienti affetti da demenza di Alzheimer]. *Neurol Psichiatr Sci Um* (Italy) 10(2): 201-15, 1990.

Chim. Actual. Alzheimer's Disease: Agreement Between Roche and Sigma-Tau. 395: 8, Nov 18, 1991.

Cipolli C and Chiari G. Effetti della L-acetilcarnitina sul deterioramento mentale dell'anziano: primi risultati [Effects of L-acetylcarnitine on mental deterioration in the aged: initial results]. *Clin Ter* 132(6 Suppl): 479-510, 31 March 1990.

Cucinotta D, Passeri M, Ventura S, Ianuccelli M, Senin U, Bonati PA and Parnetti L. Multicenter clinical placebo-controlled study with acetyl-L-carnitine (LAC) in the treatment of mildly demented elderly patients. *Drug Dev Res* (USA) 14(3-4): 213-16, 1988.

Drago F, Continella G, Pennisi G, Alloro MC, Calvani M and Scapagnini U. Behavioral effects of acetyl-L-carnitine in the male rat. *Pharmacology, Biochemistry, and Behavior* 24(5): 1393-6, 1986.

Fiore L and Rampello L. L-acetylcarnitine attenuates the age-dependent decrease of NMDA-sensitive glutamate receptors in rat hippocampus. *Acta Neurologica* 11(5): 346-50, 1989.

Franceschi C, Cossarizza A, Troiano L, Salati R and Monti D. Immunological parameters in aging: studies on natural immunomodulatory and immunoprotective substances. *Int J Clin Pharmacol Res* 10(1-2): 53-7, 1990.

Fulgente T, Onofrj M, Del Re ML, Ferracci F, Bazzano S, Ghilardi MF and Malatesta G. Laevo-acetylcarnitine (Nicetile (R)) treatment of senile depression. *Clin Trials J* (United Kingdom) 27(3): 155-63, 1990.

Garzya G, Corallo D, Fiore A, Lecciso G, Petrelli G and Zotti C. Evaluation of the effects of L-acetylcarnitine on senile patients suffering from depression. *Drugs Exp Clin Res* (Switzerland) 16(2): 101-6, 1990.

Gecele M, Francesetti G and Meluzzi A. Acetyl-L-carnitine in aged subjects with major depression: Clinical efficacy and effects on the circadian rhythm of cortisol. *Dementia* (Switzerland) 2(6): 333-7, 1991.

Ghirardi O, Caprioli A, Milano S, Giuliani A, Ramacci MT and Angelucci L. Active avoidance learning in old rats chronically treated with levocarnitine acetyl. *Physiol Behav* 52(1): 185-7, July 1992.

Ghirardi O, Giuliani A, Caprioli A, Ramacci MT and Angelucci L. Spatial memory in aged rats: population heterogeneity and effect of levocarnitine acetyl. *J Neurosci Res* 31(2): 375-9, February 1992.

Ghirardi O, Milano S, Ramacci MT, Angelucci L. Long-term acetyl-L-carnitine preserves spatial learning in the senescent rat. *Progress in Neuro-Psychopharmacology & Biological Psychiatry* 13(1-2): 237-45, 1989.

Harsing LG Jr, Sershen H, Toth E, Hashim A, Ramacci MT and Lajtha A. Acetyl-L-carnitine releases dopamine in rat corpus striatum: an *in vivo* microdialysis study. *Eur J Pharmacol* 218(1): 117-21, 21 July 1992.

Herrmann WM, Dietrich B and Hiersemenzel R. Pharmaco-electroencephalographic and clinical effects of the cholinergic substance — acetyl-L-carnitine — in patients with organic brain syndrome. *Int J Clin Pharmacol Res* 10(1-2): 81-4, 1990.

Kohjimoto Y, Ogawa T, Matsumoto M, Shirakawa K, Kuwaki T, Yasuda H, Anami K, Fujii T, Satoh H and Ono T. Effects of acetyl-L-carnitine on the brain lipofuscin content and emotional behavior in aged rats. *Japanese Journal of Pharmacology* 48, 365-71, 1988.

Laguzzi F, Moscato M, Ravera C, Bellora A, Estienne G and Coscia M. Evaluation of the efficacy of acetyl-L-carnitine in cerebral aging processes [Valutazione dell'efficacia dell'acetil-L-carnitina nei processi di invecchiamento cerebrale]. *Arch Med Interna* (Italy) 44(2): 133-36, 1992.

Lino A, Boccia MM, Rusconi AC, Bellomonte L and Cocuroccia BI. Cambiamenti psicofunzionali dello stato di vigilanza e dell'apprendimento sotto l'azione della L-acetilcarnitina in 17 giovani soggetti. Studio pilota per l'impiego nel decadimento mentale [Psycho-functional changes in attention and learning under the action of L-acetylcarnitine in 17 young subjects. A pilot study of its use in mental deterioration]. *Clin Ter* (Italy) 140(6): 569-73, June 1992.

Markowska AL and Olton DS. Dietary acetyl-L-carnitine improves spatial behaviour of old rats. *Int J Clin Pharmacol Res* 10(1-2), 65-8, 1990.

Passeri M, Cucinotta D, Bonati PA, Iannuccelli M, Parnetti L and Senin U. Acetyl-L-carnitine in the treatment of mildly demented elderly patients. *Int J Clin Pharmacol Res* 10(1-2): 75-9, 1990.

Pearson D and Shaw S. *Durk Pearson & Sandy Shaw Life Extension Newsletter* 2(10): 84-6 Jan-Feb 1990.

Postiglione A, Cicerano U, Soricelli A, De Chiara S, Gallotta G, Salvatore M and Mancini M. Cerebral blood flow in patients with chronic cerebrovascular disease: effect of acetyl L-carnitine. *Int J Clin Pharmacol Res* 10(1-2): 129-32, 1990.

Puca FM, Genco S, Specchio LM, Brancasi B, D'Ursi R, Prudenzano A, Miccoli A, Scarcia R, Martino R and Savarese M. Clinical pharmacodynamics of acetyl-L-carnitine in patients with Parkinson's disease. *Int J Clin Pharmacol Res* 10(1-2): 139-43, 1990.

Rai G, Wright G, Scott L, Beston B, Rest J and Exton-Smith AN. Double-blind, placebo controlled study of acetyl-L-carnitine in patients with Alzheimer's dementia. *Current Medical Research and Opinion* 11(10): 638-47, 1990.

Rosadini G, Marenco S, Nobili F, Novellone G and Rodriquez G. Acute effects of L-acetylcarnitine on regional cerebral blood flow in patients with cerebrovascular disease. *Clin Trials J* (United Kingdom) 25(Suppl. 1): 35-42, 1988.

Sano M, Bell K, Cote L, Dooneief G, Lawton A, Legler L, Marder K, Naini A, Stern Y and Mayeux R. Double-blind parallel design pilot study of acetyl levocarnitine in patients with Alzheimer's disease. *Arch Neurol* (United States) 49(11): 1137-41, November 1992.

Scrofani A, Biondi R, Sofia V, D'Alpa F, Grasso A and Filetti S. EEG patterns of patients with cerebrovascular damage. Effect of L-acetylcarnitine during sleep *Clin Trials J* (United Kingdom) 25(Suppl. 1): 65-71, 1988.

Sershen H, Harsing LG Jr, Banay-Schwartz M, Hashim A, Ramacci MT and Lajtha A. Effect of acetyl-L-carnitine on the dopaminergic system in aging brain. *J Neurosci Res* (USA) 30(3): 555-59, 1991.

Sinforiani E, Iannuccelli M, Mauri M, Costa A, Merlo P, Bono G and Nappi G. Neuropsychological changes in demented patients treated with acetyl-L-carnitine. *Int J Clin Pharmacol Res* 10(1-2): 69-74, 1990.

Tempesta E, Casella L, Pirrongelli C, Janiri L, Calvani M, Ancona L. L-acetylcarnitine in depressed elderly subjects. A cross-over study vs. placebo. *Drugs Under Experimental Clinical Research* 13(7): 417-23, 1987.

Tempesta E, Troncon R, Janiri L, Colusso L, Riscica P, Saraceni G, Gesmundo E, Calvani M, Benedetti N and Pola P. Role of acetyl-L-carnitine in the treatment of cognitive deficit in chronic alcoholism. *Int J Clin Pharmacol Res* 10(1-2): 101-7, 1990.

Vecchi GP, Chiari G, Cipolli C, Cortelloni C, De Vreese L and Neri M. Acetyl-L-carnitine treatment of mental impairment in the elderly: Evidence from a multicentre study. *Arch Gerontol Geriatr* (Netherlands) 12(Suppl. 2): 159-68, 1991.

Villardita C, Smirni P and Vecchio I. N-acetylcarnitine in depressed elderly patients [L'Acetil carnitina nei disturbi della sfera affettiva dell'anziano]. *Eur Rev Med Pharmacol Sci* (Italy) 6(2): 341-44, 1984.

Piracetam Update

This unique substance is probably the most popular smart drug for normal, healthy people. We've received many positive comments about piracetam in the smart-drug fan mail. Some of the most interesting of these piracetam stories (and a couple of mild caveats) are included in the Smart Drug Users chapter of this book.

In the three years since *Smart Drugs & Nutrients* was researched and published, over 150 papers have appeared in the world's scientific literature which describe human studies of piracetam. Piracetam is, in fact, a broadly effective enhancer of many

glutamic acid   pyroglutamic acid   piracetam

oxiracetam   pramiracetam

aniracetam

The Nootropic Family of Drugs and Nutrients

aspects of human performance. The studies presented in this chapter clearly indicate the breadth of piracetam's clinical application. These studies amply illustrate piracetam's benefits for normal, healthy adults, normally aging elderly adults, and people suffering from overt cognitive disorders like senility and Alzheimer's disease.

Piracetam and Weekend Athletes

The ability of piracetam to reduce metabolic stress under low-oxygen conditions was investigated by Schaffler and Klausnitzer in 1988. The researchers induced hypoxia (low oxygen levels) in healthy young men (early 20s to early 30s) by reducing the oxygen content of the laboratory air that they breathed by about half (10.5% instead of 20% oxygen). This resembled "the

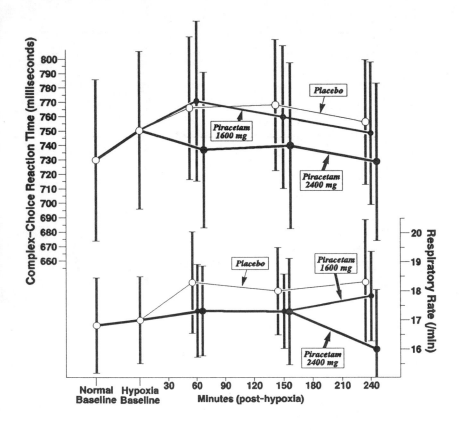

oxygen supply at an altitude of about 5300 meters" (17,400 feet). The degree of cognitive impairment due to the low oxygen levels was investigated, and the ability of piracetam (in single doses of 1600 mg or 2400 mg) to prevent this impairment was measured (see opposite figure). Half of the group was given a placebo.

Various tests of reaction time were performed, and in all cases, the piracetam-treated group performed better. Best results were obtained at the higher dose (see opposite figure, upper data points). The increased breathing rate that is usually seen under low oxygen conditions was significantly reduced by a single dose of piracetam (lower data points).

The significance of these results is that normal, healthy people who travel from lower altitudes to higher altitudes for physical activities that require stamina, coordination, concentration, and muscular output are likely to greatly benefit from piracetam. Skiers, take note! Smart-drugged skiers on vacation are probably less likely to injure themselves or someone else, and may be more likely to enjoy their vacation. Piracetam will probably not only make high-altitude sports safer, but is likely to improve performance as well.

Other high-altitude activities likely to be safer with piracetam include mountain bicycling, backpacking, rock climbing, hang gliding, and bungee jumping. And piracetam is likely to improve performance of the sport.

All of these activities involve some risk. Statistically speaking, compared to taking piracetam these sports are absolutely throw-caution-to-the-wind dare-devilish. Recently a bungee jumping trainer forgot to attach his own bungee to the mooring and jumped to his death. Would he have forgotten if he had taken piracetam? The research points to a decrease in the odds of making just this kind of error.

Piracetam for Cigarette Smokers

Of even more potential significance is the possibility that other disease conditions resulting from low oxygen levels in the blood may also be alleviated by piracetam. For example, a two-pack-per-day cigarette smoker at sea level has the oxygen levels of a person at 10,000 feet. Also, many clinical conditions like atherosclerosis (occluded arteries) and many pulmonary diseases (especially emphysema) cause reduced blood and brain oxygenation. Piracetam may greatly relieve the adverse effects of oxygen shortage in these conditions.

Driving Skills in Elderly Motorists

Statistically, middle-aged drivers have the lowest accident rates. The rate of age-related accidents can be represented by a graph with a U-shaped curve (see illustration below) with the highest values in the late teens (learning to drive) and early twenties (learning traffic judgment), the lowest values in middle age (maximum skill, experience and judgment), and higher levels again at advanced ages (impaired vision, hearing, reaction time and/or judgment).

One study of elderly drivers (average age 62.7 years) showed slightly diminished performance in "driving tasks" as compared to middle-aged drivers (average age 40.6 years). This decrement was characterized by significantly diminished performance in sign observance, lane discipline, hesitant driving, technical handling, and "junction alertness" (leading to "twice as many risk situations which required driving-instructor intervention"). No differences in speed or safe-distance behavior were noted between the groups.

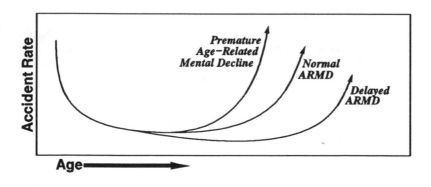

Could piracetam alter the shape of the accident curve and alleviate these decrements in older drivers by delaying the onset and slowing the progression of age-related changes?

A recent study conducted at the University of Cologne in Germany was performed to answer this question [Schmidt, 1991]. The researchers examined the driving skills of 101 elderly drivers with "reduced reaction capacity." In a randomized, double-blind, placebo-controlled study, in real-traffic conditions, those patients treated with piracetam exhibited significantly improved performance. Over the six-week test period, piracetam-treated drivers' "sign-observance" scores improved from 77.08% pre-treatment to 84.16% post-treatment.

This study indicates clearly that some of the age-related reductions in driving performance can be improved by piracetam. In only six weeks, the piracetam-treated drivers improved 7.08% on the sign-observance test. Of particular interest is the authors' note that "*all* of the drivers who scored less than 80% improved when treated with piracetam." This indicates that piracetam is most helpful in those people with the greatest driving impairment.

The number and percentage of elderly drivers in developed countries is increasing, as birth rates drop and life-expectancy increases. The extent to which widespread piracetam use by elderly drivers might diminish the rising costs of accidents caused by elderly drivers is not yet known, but it is certainly worth investigating.

Changes in Attitudes

Only three years ago, smart-drug critics were focusing on the lack of human testing in normal, healthy individuals. They said, "just because piracetam corrects cognitive deficits caused by disease doesn't mean it will correct cognitive deficits caused by aging, or that it will enhance cognitive abilities in healthy people." However, increasing data now confirm that piracetam does, in fact, improve cognitive performance in normal people.

One of the first pioneering studies to investigate this possibility was conducted 17 years ago in Sweden long before the complaints of smart-drug critics [Mindus, 1976]. These researchers selected late-middle-aged test subjects (50 years and older) of above average intelligence (their IQs averaged above 120) and who were otherwise healthy (none had any clinical signs of rapidly deteriorating mental abilities).

All 18 test subjects reported "slight but seemingly permanent reduction for some years in their capacity to retain or recall information" (AAMI). They all had developed compensatory strategies and behaviors to continue in their highly demanding jobs, such as "taking notes" and "working slower." All in all, these subjects were a good cross-section of the more productive and accomplished senior members of the work force.

The researchers employed a double-blind, cross-over study. Half of the test subjects were given placebo for the first four weeks (phase 1), and piracetam (4.8 grams daily) for the second four weeks (phase 2). The other half were given piracetam first, and placebo second.

The subjects then took a number of performance tests, including computer-based tests. In all phases of testing, piracetam scores were higher. In the cross-over phase, all subjects who switched from placebo to piracetam improved in score, and all subjects who switched from piracetam to placebo lowered in score (see the graphs below).

The computer-test results were converted into like-magnitude units to illustrate the similarity of the performance increases from piracetam. It can be seen that all five computerized tests showed identical magnitude gains. This is certainly a striking observation, given the selective effects of some other smart drugs. Piracetam and other nootropic drugs seem to produce positive effects in many aspects of mental function.

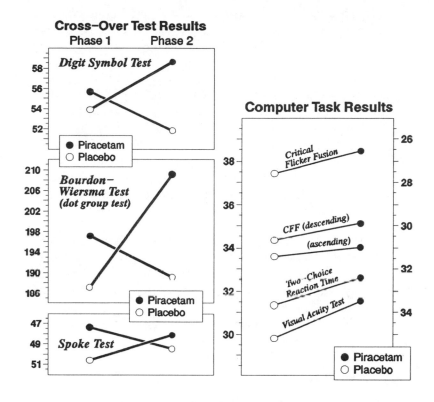

Cross–Over Test Results

Computer Task Results

Claims that smart drugs have not proven effective on normal, healthy people are clearly wrong. Such allegations are not based on science, but rather on the personal prejudices of the accusers and their unfamiliarity with the scientific literature.

Cognitive Enhancement in Senility

Although some critics may criticize the use of smart drugs to treat AAMI, many acknowledge that smart drugs *are* effective in the treatment of overt senile cognitive impairment. In a recent study of 84 geriatric patients with non-vascular senile cognitive deterioration, piracetam was found to be better than a placebo at enhancing several cognitive abilities, including attention, memory, and behavior [Fioravanti, 1991]. Dosages of 6 grams per day appeared to be more effective than 3 grams per day. However, once optimum benefits had been obtained on the 6-gram-per-day dose, the 3-gram-per-day dose was adequate to maintain the cognitive gains induced by the higher dose.

Cognitive Performance in Epileptics

Anti-epileptic medicines often exhibit cognitive side effects in the inverted-U dose-response manner. For example, at low doses, many anti-epileptic drugs improve cognition scores. However, at the high doses often necessary to control epileptic seizures, anti-epileptic drugs can cause profound cognitive impairment.

In a new study of the cognitive properties of piracetam in epileptic patients, piracetam was found to significantly improve cognitive test results without interfering with the efficacy of anti-epileptic medications. Patients taking one anti-seizure drug (carbamazepine) appeared to have even greater seizure protection when the carbamazepine was combined with piracetam [Chaudhry, 1992].

New Research Trends

Recent research into the mechanisms of nootropic drugs (drugs in the same class as piracetam) is shedding light on the crucial question, "How does piracetam work?" New findings point to a number of modes of action, including 1) stimulation of glucose metabolism, 2) increased ATP turnover, 3) increased 'internal messenger' (cyclic AMP, or cAMP) levels, 4) enhanced phospholipid levels, 5) increased protein bio-synthesis, and 6) increased cholinergic and dopaminergic stimulation. Nootropics also seem to produce resistance to several neurotoxic substances, and stimulate learning through influences on the hippocampus and cortex. Oxygen utilization by the brain appears to be significantly enhanced. [Schaffler, *et al.*, 1988].

The Recognition Piracetam Deserves

It is long past time to recognize and acknowledge that piracetam does indeed enhance cognition in both normal healthy people *and* the cognitively impaired. In 1990, piracetam sales from one brand alone (Nootropil, UCB) topped *one billion dollars* worldwide. According to UCB's annual report, Nootropil sales are still increasing, years after their patent on piracetam has expired, and numerous competitive generic piracetam products have entered the market. After decades of completely safe use, and millions of prescription and over-the-counter sales in many countries, we believe that it's time for the United States to join the rest of the world in approving piracetam for its citizens. Piracetam's absence of any known toxicity makes it an ideal candidate for over-the-counter status.

Precautions

Piracetam may increase the effects of certain drugs, such as amphetamines, psychotropics, and Hydergine, as previously stated. Adverse effects are extremely rare, but include insomnia, psychomotor agitation, nausea, gastrointestinal distress, and headaches. Piracetam has no known toxicity or contraindications.

Dosage

Piracetam is supplied in 400 mg or 800 mg capsules or tablets. The usual dose is 2400 to 4800 mg per day in three divided doses. Some literature recommends a high "attack" dose be taken for the first two days. We have noticed that often when people first take piracetam they do not notice any effect at all until they take a high dose (approximately 4000 to 8000 mg). Thereafter, they may notice that a lower dosage is sufficient. Piracetam takes effect within 30 to 60 minutes.

▷ **Note** that piracetam seems to synergize with other smart drugs. If piracetam is combined with other smart drugs, the dosage of one or more drugs/nutrients may need to be reduced.

Sources

Piracetam is not available in the U.S. but can be easily ordered from most overseas mail-order pharmacies. An up-to-date listing of such overseas sources is maintained by CERI (see the tearout card at the front of this book).

References

Chaudhry HR, Najam N, De Mahieu C, Raza A, Ahmad N. Clinical use of piracetam in epileptic patients. *Curr Ther Res Clin Exp* 52(3): 355-60, 1992.

Fioravanti M, Bergamasco B, Bocola V, *et al.*. A multicentre, double-blind, controlled study of piracetam vs. placebo in geriatric patients with nonvascular mild-moderate impairment in cognition. *New Trends in Clinical Neuropharmacology* (Italy) 5(1): 27-34, 1991.

Mindus P, Cronholm B, Levander SE, and Schalling D. Piracetam-induced study on normally aging individuals. *Acta Psychiat Scand* 54: 150-60, 1976.

Schaffler K and Klausnitzer W. Randomized placebo-controlled double-blind cross-over study on antihypoxidotic effects of piracetam using psychophysiological measures in healthy volunteers. *Arzneim-Forsch* 38(2): 288-91, 1988.

Schmidt U, Brendemuhl D, Engels K, *et al.*. Arbeits und Forschungsgemeinschaft fur Strassenverkehr und Verkehrssicherheit. *Pharmacopsychiatry* (Germany) 24(4): 121-26, July 1991.

Vitamin Update

When *Smart Drugs & Nutrients* was written in 1990, vitamins were still considered "fringe science" by many in the medical profession. Nevertheless, we reviewed in that book some of the scientific evidence on the cognitive-performance-enhancing benefits of vitamins.

Since the publication of *Smart Drugs & Nutrients*, there seems to have been a paradigm shift away from the bad old days of physicians warning against vitamins, to a new consensus in the scientific and medical community that vitamins are potent disease fighters and potential aging-retardants.

On April 6, 1992, *Time* magazine published a cover story on vitamins, proclaiming that, "New evidence shows they may help fight cancer, heart disease, and the ravages of aging." A mere ten years ago, such a story would have generated a storm of protest from medical authorities. Today, the ever-mounting evidence for the abilities of nutrients to prevent and treat disease is so overwhelming that only a few die-hard anti-vitamin medical "authorities" remain vocal critics. Vitamins are now mainstream.

As Barbara Walters commented on ABC's *Nightline*, "There was a time when doctors said, 'Eat a balanced diet and you don't have to take vitamins.' Now we are learning that this vitamin or that vitamin might help prevent cancer." At the 1992 *American Aging Association* Conference in San Francisco, one researcher volunteered that nearly everyone in the field of gerontology (the study of aging) is now taking megadoses of vitamins. Ten years ago, only a few were.

Approximately half of all Americans take vitamin supplements and about half of those take daily supplements. Americans spend $3.3 billion on vitamins and nutrients every year — and that figure is growing.

Smarter School Children

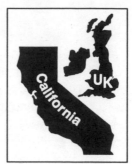

In 1988, a California research team headed by Dr. Stephen Schoenthaler and the English research team of Benton and Roberts both found that simple vitamin supplementation of schoolchildren produced non-verbal IQ increases of an average of six points (see illustration below). The near-simultaneous release of these near-identical findings garnered international headlines. In England, the publicity triggered a buying enthusiasm that stripped many store shelves of vitamin supplements in days. It is estimated that 80-150 million pounds Sterling (up to 300 million U.S. dollars) was spent in one week, and this by a population only twice that of the state of California.

In 1991, Dr. Schoenthaler and colleagues replicated their earlier study with an expanded study of 615 school children from a half-dozen schools (with varied socioeconomic profiles) in Stanislaus County, California. The children were randomly assigned to one of four different groups that received various vitamin-mineral supplements or placebo on a triple-blind basis (the students, testers and scientists did not know to which group each student had been assigned). The 12-week study was designed to more precisely quantify the *degree* of IQ

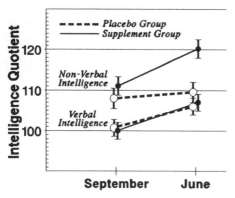

Intelligence Increases in Schoolchildren

Over the course of a school year, supplemented students gained 9 non-verbal IQ points while control students gained 2 points. This is a net gain of 7 IQ points. Verbal IQ scores were essentially similar in both groups: a gain of 7 points in the supplemented students compared to 5 for the control students [Schoenthaler, 1988].

enhancement and to determine whether the intelligence increases seen in the earlier studies were due to a general effect on most children, or to effects on a smaller subset of children (presumably suffering from some kinds of sub-clinical nutritional deficiencies). The first test group received only a placebo. The second group received a 50% RDA supplement (designed to bring nutritional status up to minimal RDA levels). The third group was given a 100% RDA supplement, and the fourth a 200% supplement (of most, but not all, vitamins and minerals — see table below).

Supplement Formulas Used in California Schoolchildren IQ Study

Vitamin/Mineral	Group 2 "50% RDA"		Group 3 "100% RDA"		Group 4 "200% RDA"	
Vitamin A	2500 IU	50%	5000 IU	100%	5000 IU	100%
Vitamin B_1 (thiamine)	0.75 mg	50%	1.7 mg	100%	3.4 mg	200%
Vitamin B_2 (riboflavin)	0.85 mg	50%	1.7 mg	100%	3.4 mg	200%
Vitamin B_3 (niacin)	10 mg	50%	20 mg	100%	40 mg	200%
Vitamin B_5 (pantothenate)	5 mg	50%	10 mg	100%	20 mg	200%
Vitamin B_6 (pyridoxine)	1 mg	50%	2 mg	100%	4 mg	200%
Vitamin B_{12}	3 mcg	50%	6 mcg	100%	12 mcg	200%
Vitamin C	30 mg	50%	60 mg	100%	120 mg	200%
Vitamin D	200 I.U.	50%	400 I.U.	100%	400 I.U.	100%
Vitamin E	15 I.U.	50%	30 I.U.	100%	60 I.U.	200%
Vitamin K	50 mcg	*	50 mcg	*	50 mcg	*
Biotin	150 mcg	50%	300 mcg	100%	300 mcg	100%
Folic Acid	200 mcg	50%	400 mcg	100%	400 mcg	100%
Calcium	200 mg	20%	200 mg	20%	200 mg	20%
Chromium	50 mcg	*	100 mcg	*	200 mcg	*
Copper	1 mg	50%	2 mg	100%	3 mg	150%
Iodine	75 mcg	50%	150 mcg	100%	150 mcg	100%
Iron	9 mg	50%	18 mg	100%	36 mg	200%
Magnesium	80 mg	20%	80 mg	20%	80 mg	20%
Manganese	1.25 mg	*	2.5 mg	*	5 mg	*
Molybdenum	120 mcg	*	250 mcg	*	500 mcg	*
Selenium	50 mcg	*	100 mcg	*	200 mcg	*
Zinc	7.5 mg	50%	15 mg	100%	30 mg	200%

* The U.S. RDA has not been established for these essential nutrients [Schoenthaler, et al., 1991].

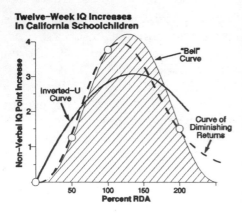

Twelve-Week IQ Increases
In California Schoolchildren

IQ Increases vs Dosage
Results of Schoenthaler and colleagues' 1991 study of IQ. The results (open circles) suggest an inverted-U dose-response curve for vitamin supplementation. They can be fitted to a "bell" shaped curve (shaded area) or to a curve of diminishing returns (dashed line). Larger studies will be required to accurately assign the dose-response curve with certainty.

The 100% RDA group scored a 3.7-point relative increase in the non-verbal IQ scores during the 12-week period. The 50% and 200% groups experienced smaller but significant relative increases of 1.2 and 1.5 points, respectively (see illustration above).

These results suggest that vitamins may also have an inverted-U-shaped dose-response curve like most of the other cognition-enhancing drugs. This study suggests that optimum intake in adolescents might be between one and two times the RDA (see illustration above).

Not every child in the study experienced an increased IQ with nutritional supplementation. One-third, however, experienced a dramatic *ten-point jump* in IQ. These results suggest that a significant proportion of "normal, healthy" children are in fact *sub-clinically nutritionally deficient*, even though they show no overt signs of physiological pathology. The data validate the earlier findings of Sandstead [1986] and Cherkin [1987], which suggest that mental dysfunction is one of the first manifestations of nutritional deficiency.

In an exclusive interview with *Smart Drug News*, the principal investigator of the study, Dr. Schoenthaler, stated:

> *"The IQ difference between an average American and a doctor, lawyer, or professor is only about 11 points. The*

*gain observed in one out of three [study participants] is
the same as might be required for an average American to
aspire to be a doctor, lawyer or professor."*

Is this a substantial benefit? What do you think? Should this
approach be incorporated into our national education policy?
With academic performance test scores on the decline, one
might assume that professional educators and government
agencies would be rushing to get with the program. Alas, not
so. Educators are looking for teaching solutions, not nutritive
ones. And government bureaucrats are terrorized by the
possibility that declining quality of nutrition might be
responsible for declining test scores. Increasing nutritional
standards by improving the quality of *food* would cost many
billions in federal lunch programs and other entitlements.
Using low-cost supplements would require formal government
recognition of the benefits of vitamin supplements and an open
acknowledgement of the poor nutritional quality of foods in
general, an idea completely against both FDA policy and
orthodox medical dogma.

Fortunately, vitamin supplements do not require public policy.
Individual students and their parents can opt to partake of
vitamin supplements without the sanction or approval of
governmental regulatory agencies. At least they can right now.
Next year may be different (see the Health Freedom Struggle
section). For more details on Dr. Schoenthaler's program, read
his book, *Improve Your Child's IQ and Behavior*, published by
BBC Books, Woodland's 80, Wood Lane, London W12 0TT,
United Kingdom.

Teenagers, Violence and Vitamins

Dr. Schoenthaler's latest study may have equally profound
implications for society. Working with over 400 of the most
violent teenagers incarcerated by the California Youth
Authority, Schoenthaler and colleagues have administered
vitamins and placebo on a triple-blind basis. That means that
no one, including the researchers, knew which adolescents were
receiving vitamins.

At the time of this writing, the results have not been published. However, Schoenthaler hints that this study will replicate his earlier findings in a similar, smaller study conducted in an Oklahoma juvenile correctional facility in 1988. That study found that the group taking vitamins had an *immediate* 50% reduction in violence. The vitamin-supplemented group showed great reductions in the incidence of "hyperkinesis, hyperactivity, insubordination, fighting, truancy, and assault and battery." In his interview, Dr. Schoenthaler summarized these findings:

"We basically cut the violence, the antisocial behavior, hyperactivity, and all types of rule violations in half. While the placebo group did show some improvement, the massive improvement was seen only in the supplement group. We examined multiple measures of behavior — for example, how often children attacked each other, how often they attacked staff members, how often they got in trouble at the correctional-facility school, and the rate of injuries from the attacks — every way we could validate serious violence. The improvement in behavior was coming from the supplement group, and the entire institution was running much smoother as a result — all of this from an improvement in nutrition!"

When we suggested that the cost of running that institution might be dramatically lowered by this change, Schoenthaler surprised us by agreeing — and added:

"The staff decided for itself that the improvement was too important to wait for the state government to decide the long-term policy implications of the results. The improvement took place virtually overnight — within 48 hours, it chopped the rate of violence in half. Rather than go back to the way it was before the study started, the institutional staff pooled their money and bought supplements for the kids instead of waiting for the state to eventually take action."

You read that correctly. Oklahoma state employees, *out of their own pockets*, paid for vitamins for the institutionally incarcerated children! When we asked if anyone has done an informal economic analysis of the savings that might be gained with this kind of program, Dr. Schoenthaler told us:

> *"It's been done several times. The savings from the use of supplements can be astronomical. The cost of giving these supplements to an incarcerated delinquent for a year, depending on the caliber of what one uses and the wholesale cost, varies from a low of $15 to a high of $30-$40 per person. The cost to keep them locked up is about $36,000 per child per year. The violence is a significant fraction of that total cost. The violence results in a lot of medical bills and lawsuits. The average cost of one of these court cases runs $6000-$7000."*

He summarized, "If you look at your ratio of the savings to the cost of vitamin supplementation, it is 100 to 1, or 1000 to 1." Even ignoring the benefits to the children and staff members, economic savings alone make implementation of this application of smart nutrients attractive.

Smart Nutrient Conclusions

These research findings with vitamins and IQ, and with vitamins and violence, are not exactly new. Earlier studies have identified such learning and behavioral benefits from improvements in *food quality*. The problem with the earlier studies is that improved food quality brought not only improved nutritional values, but improved *attention from staff*. Were the kids responding to the nutrients or to the attention? Until the double-blind (or triple-blind) studies with supplements eliminated the attention factor, we couldn't know for sure. Now that we have, we know for sure. Improved nutrition means improved learning. Improved nutrition means better behavior. It's time to use this technology. All of our schools can use less violence.

The Health Freedom Struggle

At the time of this writing (June 15, 1993), vitamins, minerals, amino acids and herbs are readily available over the counter in the United States. By the time you read this, this may have changed. In 1992, the FDA submitted thousands of pages of regulations for the Nutritional Labeling and Education Act (NLEA). With the NLEA, the FDA gave itself the power to remove all amino acids, herbs, and above-RDA vitamins from the U.S. market. The NLEA was originally scheduled to become law in May of 1993, but massive consumer outcry prompted Congress to pass a moratorium on the NLEA in the last days of the 1992 session. The moratorium postponed enforcement of the NLEA until December of 1993. The FDA's hands were effectively tied for the year.

The Health Freedom Acts

Attempts to retain over-the-counter access to amino acids, herbs and high-potency vitamins have been focused on getting health-freedom legislation through Congress. This legislation was written to prevent the FDA from classifying supplements as drugs.

The first such bill was the Health Freedom Act of 1992 introduced by Senator Orrin Hatch. If the Health Freedom Act had passed, companies would have been allowed to make any *truthful* medical claim about a supplement, as long as there was "reasonable" scientific evidence for that claim. The FDA would have been barred from classifying dietary supplements as drugs (and requiring costly FDA approval).

In February of 1993, a nearly identical act (The Health Freedom Act of 1993) was introduced by Representative Elton Gallegly of California. Two months later, two Dietary Supplement Health and Education Acts (DSHEA) were introduced — one in the Senate by Orrin Hatch, and one in the House by Bill Richardson. At the time of this writing, all three bills have yet to be voted on. Subscribe to *Smart Drug News* to

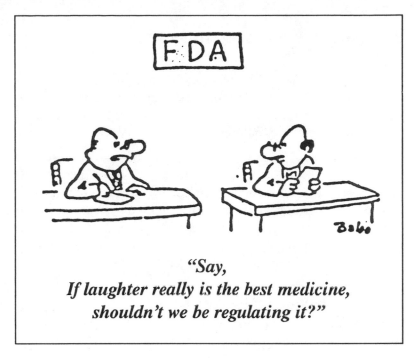

"Say,
If laughter really is the best medicine,
shouldn't we be regulating it?"

stay up-to-date with this rapidly developing issue (see the tearout card at the front of the book).

When legislation such as the Health Freedom Act finally does pass (if it does), we will see a revolution in medicine and health care. Pharmaceutical companies will have the choice to continue doing what they are doing now (developing new, patentable drugs for which they can make *one* claim after going through a 10-year, $200 million approval process) or they can develop and market natural products and make hundreds of legal, *truthful* health claims. Good business sense will favor the latter. Once nutrient claims are no longer censored by the FDA, competition between drugs and nutrients will likely favor the lower-cost, lower-toxicity dietary supplements. Pharmaceutical companies may decide to buy up some of the small and medium-sized supplement companies as they move into this new and exciting area of medicine.

The Health Insurance Industry to the Rescue?

We hope that sometime in the near future, some CEO or other big-wig in the medical insurance industry may notice that the FDA's prohibition on truthful claims about vitamins is costing the insurance industry billions of dollars every year.

Think about it. If every label on every bottle of vitamin C included the truthful claim, "In a recent study of over 11,000 people, men who took more than 600 mg of vitamin C per day lived 6 years longer than those taking minimal vitamin C," more men would be taking vitamin C, correct? Those men will live longer and require less health care than those not taking vitamin C. They will make more insurance payments and file fewer claims.

If insurance industry CEOs and their lobbyists in Washington start calling the appropriate Senators and Representatives, then we will have health freedom in the U.S. Compared to the medical insurance industry, the FDA is small potatoes.

Four Out of Five FDA Researchers Take Vitamins

Although the FDA has a clear anti-vitamin bias, not everybody working for the agency agrees with this policy. At a recent conference on aging, five FDA researchers in attendance stated that they were all using megadoses of vitamins for disease prevention. Four of the five added that they believed the vitamins would provide life-extension benefits as well. Paradigm shift indeed.

Vitamins and the Elderly

Nowhere is the issue of vitamins and cognitive function more applicable than with the elderly. The overall quality of life for the elderly is largely determined by their general health, capacity for mobility, and mental function. With good health, mobility and mental alertness, perceptions of independence and feelings of self-esteem are high. With disease, infirmity, and mental decline comes dependence, feelings of helplessness and inadequacy, and diminished self-esteem. Many of these age-associated physical and mental declines are known to be closely related to quality of nutrition.

Adequate vitamin D and magnesium intakes are needed for maintenance of muscle capacity [Fiatarone, 1990]. High vitamin C protects against cataract formation. And adequate intakes of vitamins B_{12}, B_6 and folic acid are critical for cognitive function.

As an example of the kind of epidemiological findings relating nutrition to health, one study found that those people in the lowest 25% for vitamin C intake had 3.7 times higher incidence of central cataract and 14 times higher incidence of posterior

Possible Neurological Effects of Specific Vitamin Deficiencies	
Vitamin	**Manifestation**
Thiamine (B_1)	Beri-beri, Wernicke-Korsakoff psychosis.
Riboflavin (B_2)	Cognitive impairment, memory deficit.
Niacin (vitamin B_3)	Pellagra, dementia, rage syndrome.
Pantothenic acid (B_5)	Myelin degeneration.
Pyridoxine (B_6)	Convulsions, peripheral neuropathy.
Cobalamin (B_{12})	Dementia, peripheral neuropathy, subacute combined system degeneration, cognitive impairment, memory deficit, depression, paresthesia, ataxia, mood disturbances, delusions, paranoia.
Folic acid (folate)	Irritability, depression, paranoia, cognitive impairment, memory deficit, forgetfulness, EEG abnormalities, dementia, epilepsy, schizophrenia.
Vitamin C (ascorbate)	Cognitive impairment, memory deficit.
Vitamin E (tocopherol)	Peripheral axonopathy, spinocereballar degeneration.

subcapsular cataract than those in the highest 25% for vitamin C intake [Jacques, 1988]. The relationship between high intakes of other antioxidants like vitamin E (tocopherol) and beta-carotene and reduced cataract incidence is also substantial.

Decreased intakes of almost any essential nutrient adversely influences the immune system — especially cellular immunity. In studies of elderly people, supplemental vitamin E and zinc have enhanced immune cell function and restored aspects of immunity to more youthful levels.

Nutrition and Cognition

Deficiencies of almost any nutrient can cause impaired nervous system function. The numerous mental and neurological manifestations of nutrient deficiencies are listed in the table below. What is not so well-established, however, is the degree to which marginal nutrient intake contributes to subclinical cognitive impairment. Widely dismissed with ridicule twenty years ago, this possibility is now receiving serious scientific consideration.

The common deficiencies of vitamin B_{12}, folic acid, and vitamin B_6 in the elderly combine to seriously impair certain of the body's enzymes. This affliction is believed to be responsible for much of the mental impairment observed in elderly individuals. It is also easily corrected through nutritional supplements.

Deficiencies of hydrochloric acid (HCl) production in the stomach are known to impair B_{12} and folic acid absorption. Up to 30% of people age 65 and older experience seriously diminished HCl production. The elderly typically exhibit diminished blood levels of folic acid and B_{12}. Furthermore, adding HCl to their diet normalizes folic acid absorption.

Nutrient deficiencies may be more difficult to recover from than to induce. The RDA of vitamin B_6, for example, is not sufficient to restore B_6 levels in the vitamin B_6-deficient elderly. This possibility was not taken into consideration when the RDAs were established.

Dr. Masaki Imagawa [1990], of the Neuropsychiatric Clinic, Amagasaki Hospital, Hyogo, Japan, evaluated the effects of vitamin B_6 and Coenzyme Q_{10} on ten patients with Alzheimer's Disease, all of whom had been unresponsive to previous therapy with vasodilators. Both substances were used in doses of 60-120 mg per day. Improvement was noted on several Alzheimer's evaluation scales (Hasagawa's Dementia Score, and the Modified Miyasaki's ADL Scale).

Magnesium as a Smart Nutrient?

Magnesium, in particular, seems to have a profound effect on dementias of various types. Dr. J. Leslie Glick [1990a, 1990b] of the Bionix Corporation reviewed the effects of 1000 mg of magnesium in patients with Alzheimer's disease and other dementias. He reports that magnesium in these doses "may improve memory and alleviate other symptoms in patients with various dementias."

By competing with calcium for ion transport, magnesium may act similarly to calcium-channel blocking drugs like nimodepine (see Nimodepine chapter). Both magnesium and nimodepine have been reported to enhance cognitive abilities. Additionally, both cause vascular dilation and are known to have anti-anxiety and anti-seizure effects.

We highly recommend magnesium supplementation to everybody. Several studies show that magnesium is one of the most common dietary deficiencies in the modern world and it is very often deficient in older people. Furthermore, there has been much speculation that magnesium deficiency may have some causal involvement with Alzheimer's disease [Borella, *et al.*, 1990; Costello, *et al.*, 1992; Durlach, 1990; Glick, 1990a, 1990b].

Magnesium comes in many forms including: magnesium oxide powder, magnesium hydroxide (milk of magnesia), magnesium carbonate, and others. There is much controversy over which form of magnesium might be the most readily absorbed and utilized by the body. In our opinion, amino-acid chelates of magnesium (such as magnesium aspartate or magnesium glycinate) are the best form for absorption.

Precautions (Vitamin Toxicity?)

The FDA has traditionally claimed that amino acids, herbs and high-potency vitamins are toxic. The FDA states that it is "concerned about the safety of food-based products such as amino acids and vitamins." But is their claim truthful?

As a physician who prescribes drugs as well as supplements, I [WD] have seen many more adverse reactions from prescription drugs than I have from non-prescription natural substances. A report by Loomis [1992] supports this observation (see following table). The table is based on data obtained from annual reports of the American Association of Poison Control Centers and summarizes the relative safety of drugs versus vitamins. Since 1983, there has been *only one* vitamin-related death. On the other hand, there were more than 2500 deaths due to several common categories of

Fatalities from Prescription Drugs, Non-Prescription Drugs, and Nutrients

	83	84	85	86	87	88	89	90	Total
Number of centers reporting	16	47	56	57	63	64	70	72	
Analgesics (pain killers)	22	53	87	82	93	118	126	134	715
Antidepressants (mood elevators)	19	57	90	100	105	135	140	159	805
Asthma Therapies	4	10	11	21	16	27	34	37	160
Cardiovascular Drugs[1]	5	18	21	50	52	65	70	79	360
Sedatives and Hypnotics[2]	11	51	62	61	48	77	78	72	460
Deaths from Amphetamines[3]	1	4	6	11	11	12	5	6	56
Deaths from all above drugs	62	193	227	325	325	434	453	487	2506
Deaths attributed to all nutrients	0	0	0	0	1[†]	0	0	1	2[†]

1. Includes blood pressure medications. 2. Includes sleeping pills and tranquilizers. 3. Includes stimulants. †The 1987 vitamin-related death report was later determined to be an error. Table adapted from Donald Loomis, *Townsend Letter for Doctors*, April 1992. Original data from the American Association of Poison Control Centers. Statistics first published in the *American Journal of Emergency Medicine.*

prescription and over-the-counter medications during the same period.

The FDA's exaggeration of nutrient toxicity borders on the ludicrous. They assert that "even ordinary nutrients such as vitamins and amino acids can be *highly toxic*" [italics ours], but the facts speak differently. One of the "toxic" amino acids that the FDA is especially concerned about is arginine. Typically used in 3-10 gram doses by consumers, arginine is administered in 30 gram *intravenous* doses by physicians *to children.* How can 10 gram self-administered oral doses be dangerous for adults while 30 gram physician-administered intravenous doses are safe in small children? This is *FDAspeak* at its most eloquent.

Certainly, isolated cases of mild adverse reactions can be found to *anything* — including aspirin, Tylenol, cold medications, appetite-suppression drugs, allergy formulas, milk, honey, Nutrasweet, herbs, niacin, zinc, salt, and even water. However, the lack of reported adverse reactions (despite the FDA's tireless efforts to encourage physicians to report such adverse reactions) to even "megadoses" of vitamins and amino acids confirms that they are *not* "highly toxic." Even tryptophan, which the FDA claims is toxic, isn't. Prior to several bad batches (manufactured by Showa Denko) that were imported into the United States, there had been *no toxicity* reported from tryptophan use — despite the fact that *14 million users* took tryptophan regularly over a *twenty-year period.*

The FDA's assertion that nutrients, amino acids, and vitamins are "highly toxic" — even with tryptophan — is just an empty, hysterical claim, without scientific merit.

Quite the contrary, the FDA's *Talk Paper* on smart drugs *confirms* that "no injuries" have so far been reported to the FDA by physicians, government agencies, or consumers for the over-100,000 estimated smart-drug users in this country. How can amino acids and vitamins be toxic when amino-acid-containing and vitamin-containing smart drinks are not causing any toxicity?

The FDA's knowledge of toxicity is appalling. A review of the available world literature on the toxicity of vitamins, amino acids and nutrients clearly indicates that the FDA is completely off base.

FDA claims of supplement toxicity are grossly exaggerated. Its censorship of truthful claims is repressive. And its intended prohibitions of amino acids, herbs and high-potency vitamins is a serious threat to public health. By its obstructionist attitudes and policies — rather than protecting the health of the American public — the FDA has become the greatest single impediment to medical progress in this country.

Sources

Please see Appendix A for a listing of sources for high-quality supplements. You can also send in the tearout card at the front of this book to get an up-to-date product sources list.

References

Benton D and Roberts G. Effect of vitamin and mineral supplementation on intelligence of a sample of schoolchildren. *The Lancet*, 23 January 1988.

Bonke D, and Nickel B. Improvement of fine motoric movement control by elevated dosages of vitamin B1, B6 and B12 in target shooting. *International Journal for Vitamins and Nutrition*: Research Supplement 30: 198-204, 1989.

Borella P, Giardino A, Neri M and Andermarker E. Magnesium and potassium status in elderly subjects with and without dementia of the Alzheimer type. *Magnes Res* 3(4): 283-9, December 1990.

Cherkin A. Interaction of nutritional factors with memory processing. In: Essman, W. (Ed.), *Nutrition and Brain Function*. Basel, Switzerland, Karger Press, 1987.

Costello RB and Moser-Veillon PB. A review of magnesium intake in the elderly. A cause for concern? *Magnes Res* 5(1): 61-7, March 1992.

Durlach J. Magnesium depletion and pathogenesis of Alzheimer's disease. *Magnes Res* 3(3): 217-8, September 1990.

Enstrom, *et al.* Vitamin C intake and mortality among a sample of the United States population. *Epidemiology* 3: 194-202, 1992.

FDA Drug Bulletin, Washington, DC.

Fiatarone MA, Marks EC, Ryan DN, *et al.* High-intensity strength training in nonagenarians. *JAMA* 263: 3029-34, 1990.

Glick LJ. Dementia: The role of magnesium deficiency and an hypothesis concerning the pathogenesis of Alzheimer's Disease. *Medical Hypotheses*, 31: 211-25, 1990a.

Glick LJ. Use of magnesium in the management of dementias. *Med Sci Res*, 18: 831-833, 1990b.

Imagawa M. Megavitamin therapy (Coenzyme Q_{10} and vitamin B_6) in Alzheimer's disease and senile dementia of Alzheimer type. In: *Basic, Clinical and Therapeutic Aspects of Alzheimer's and Parkinson's Diseases*, Volume 2, by Nagatsu, *et al.*, pp. 489-491, Plenum Press, New York, 1990.

Jacques PF, Hartx SC, Chylack LT, *et al.* Nutritional status in persons with and without senile cataract. *Am J Clin Nutr* 48: 152-8, 1988.

Loomis D. Which is safer: Drugs or vitamins? *Townsend Letter for Doctors* 219: April 1992.

Rosenberg IH and Miller JW. Nutritional factors in physical and cognitive functions of elderly people. *Am J Clin Nutr* 55: 1237S-43S, 1992.

Sandstead H. Nutrition and brain function: trace elements. *Nutrition Review* 44, 37-41, 1986.

Schoenthaler SJ, Amos SP, Eysenck HJ, Peritz E and Yudkin J. Controlled trial of vitamin-mineral supplementation: Effects on intelligence and performance. *Personality and Individual Differences* 12(4): 351-62, 1991.

Schoenthaler SJ. Diet and IQ. *Nature* 352: 292, 1991.

Suggested Treatment Protocol for Alzheimer's Disease

The primary focus for *Smart Drugs & Nutrients* and this book is the use of cognition-enhancing substances for normal people wanting to improve their brain power and prevent or treat age-associated memory impairment. However, we know that many patients suffering from Alzheimer's disease also benefit from many of the substances we discuss. We have received many gratifying reports from the families of Alzheimer's patients, and from the sufferers themselves, about the relief obtained through the use of various combinations of smart drugs and nutrients.

Alzheimer's disease is considered to be the *number one health problem* by the National Institute on Aging [Goldsmith, 1984]. Alzheimer's disease attacks between 2% and 6% of people over the age of 65. It is more common in women than in men, and there appears to be a genetic predisposition to being afflicted. The likelihood of a close relative of an Alzheimer's patient developing the disease is about four times greater than the general population. If the onset is after age 65, the average course of the disease from onset to death is about five years, with a general range of one to ten years. The duration is somewhat longer if the onset is before age 65. Three characteristics of Alzheimer's disease are: 1) severe cognitive impairment, 2) its onset and course are insidious and progressive, and 3) the diagnosis is one of *exclusion* (*i.e.*, no other discernible causes of dementia can be determined) [Cohen, 1981].

What Causes Alzheimer's Disease?

The problem with finding a cure for Alzheimer's disease is that the cause has not been determined. Scientists have made a number of educated guesses as to the cause(s), and have identified a number of contributing factors. First, as noted above, there appears to be a genetic component to Alzheimer's disease. Other suspected causes include free radical damage, slow viruses, reduced blood flow to the brain, immune system malfunction, abnormal calcium regulation within nerve cells, hormonal factors which adversely effect brain cell functioning (both too much and too little of specific hormones), malnutrition, and toxic levels of aluminum, lead and iron. All of the above factors have been implicated at one time or another as potential contributory causes of Alzheimer's disease. In fact, there may not be a *single* cause of this disease. If this is the case, there is probably not going to be a single treatment that will work for everyone. Thus, treatment modalities should be developed which approach Alzheimer's disease by attacking as many of the most likely causes that can be identified.

Another approach to treatment is to correct the biochemical and physiological changes which characterize the disease. The most widely held theory of the cause of Alzheimer's disease is the *cholinergic theory* [Drachman and Glosser, 1981]. This theory attributes the cognitive deficits of Alzheimer's disease to a breakdown in the cholinergic neurotransmitter system. Contributions by other neurotransmitter systems have also been implicated by other researchers. Thus, a useful therapeutic approach would be to 1) identify the neurotransmitter systems involved, 2) prevent their breakdown, 3) enhance sensitivity of the nerve endings to the neurotransmitters, and 4) restore normal (or *supernormal*, if necessary) levels of the neurotransmitters.

Prevention

The most cost-effective, least invasive way to treat any illness is to prevent it in the first place. Aluminum has been frequently implicated as a primary cause of Alzheimer's disease. We therefore recommend that all sources of aluminum ingestion be eliminated. This includes disposing of all aluminum cookware, avoiding beverages and foods which come in aluminum cans, not using aluminum-containing deodorants and anti-perspirants, and not taking aluminum- containing antacids and aluminum-buffered aspirin. Some cities treat drinking water with aluminum compounds that have been implicated in the incidence of Alzheimer's disease. Many water filter manufacturers advertise that their products remove aluminum.

We highly recommend the book, *Reducing the Risk of Alzheimer's Disease*, by Dr. Michael A. Weiner. This book not only provides comprehensive brand-name sources of aluminum-containing products, but also provides comprehensive preventive nutritional recommendations. It is available from Dr. Weiner at 415-388-1006.

Dr. Robert Sapolsky, of Stanford University, believes that brain cell loss in aging and Alzheimer's disease may be due to high levels of cortisol, a hormone which increases when we are under stress. He therefore recommends that efforts be made to minimize stressors in the lives of Alzheimer's disease patients. He also believes that corticosteroids should *not* be used in Alzheimer's disease patients for other medical problems like asthma or arthritis [Sapolsky and McEwen, 1986].

Importance of Early Intervention

Since loss of brain cells is a characteristic of Alzheimer's disease, it is clear that any therapeutic approach must be initiated early in the disease. Although the regrowth and regeneration of brain cells is under investigation by many different research teams around the world, no clinical therapy is yet available. Loss of brain cells must be considered permanent, and prevented whenever possible. Early intervention is essential.

Treatment Approaches

Most Alzheimer's disease clinicians and researchers concede that there is no single drug that will alleviate this condition, and that *a multiple-drug approach will be required*. We agree that a multi-pronged attack on Alzheimer's disease is necessary. This

Table 1: Recommended Combination-Therapies for Alzheimer's Disease

Substances	Dosages	Therapeutic effects	References
Thiamine (B1)	50-500 mg 3 times daily	Nutrition adjunct	Hoffer, 1993
Niacin (B3)	100-500 mg 3 times daily	Enhanced cerebral circulation Nutritional adjunct	LaBrecque & Goldberg, 1967 Loriaux, et al., 1985 Hoffer, 1993
Pyridoxine (B6)	20-60 mg 3 times daily	Support of methylation metabolism Co-factor in neurotransmitter synthesis	Imagawa, 1990 Deijen, et al., 1992
Cobalamin (B12)	1 mg weekly (by injection) or 1 mg daily (by mouth)	Age-associated loss of intrinsic factor Support of methylation metabolism	Shaw, et al., 1971 Roberts, 1982
Folic acid	5 mg daily	Support of methylation metabolism	Shaw, et al., 1971 Hoffer, 1993
Vitamin B-complex	100% RDA 3-4 times daily	Metabolic support Correction of nutritional deficiencies	Whitman, 1966 Altman, et al., 1973
Lecithin (high phosphatidylcholine) or Choline chloride	10 grams daily 3 grams daily	Membrane stabilization Acetylcholine precursor Acetylcholine precursor	Etienne, 1981 Thal, et al., 1981
DMAE or Centrophenoxine	100-1000 mg daily 600 mg 2 times daily	Precursor for choline and acetylcholine Lipofuscin removal Cholinergic enhancement Lipofuscin removal	Fisman, et al., 1981 Ferris, 1981 Ferris, 1981 Gedye, et al., 1972
Ascorbate (vitamin C)	500 mg 3 times daily up to 2000 mg 12X daily (up to bowel tolerance)	Nutritional support Water-soluble antioxidant support Sulfhydryl-reducing agent	Altman, et al., 1973 Roberts, 1982 Hoffer, 1993
Vitamin E	400-1000 IU daily	Antioxidant Lipid-membrane stabilization	Roberts, 1982

	Dosage	Action	References
Glutathione and/or **Cysteine**	100-1000 mg daily / 500-1500 mg daily	Sulfhydryl antioxidant / Sulfhydryl antioxidant and glutathione precursor	Roberts, 1982 / Fowkes, 1993
CoEnzyme Q10	60-180 mg daily	Support of energy metabolism	Imagawa, 1990 / Imagawa, et al., 1990 / Roberts, 1982
Zinc (preferably as zinc aspartate)	25 mg daily	Immune enhancement / Nutritional support	Czerwinski, et al., 1974 / Constantinidis, 1990a, 1990b
Magnesium	500 mg 2 times daily	Nutritional support / Calcium-channel inhibition	Glick, 1990a, 1990b / Landfield, 1986
Acetyl-L-carnitine	1000 mg 2-3 times daily	Cerebral metabolic enhancement	see SDII
Aspirin	300 mg daily	Anti-clotting agent / Anti-inflammatory agent	Hoffer, 1993
Deprenyl	5 mg twice daily (breakfast and lunch)	Dopaminergic neuroprotection / Neuroendocrine regulation	Knoll, 1989 / Dilman and Dean, 1992
Diapid (vasopressin) (and DDAVP)	2-3 times daily	Neuropeptide neurostimulation	Laczi, et al., 1982 / Durso, et al. 1982
DHEA	1 gram daily	Steroid precursor / Cyclic GMP stimulation	Bonnet and Brown, 1992 / Roberts, 1990
Estrogen (for women)	0.5-1.0 mg per day, days 1-25	Hormone replacement	Fillit, et al., 1986
Ginkgo biloba	40-120 mg 3 times daily	Cerebral metabolic enhancement / Cerebral circulation enhancement	see SD&N references
Hydergine	6-12 mg daily (divided doses)	Neural metabolic enhancement	see SD&N references / Kugler, et al., 1978

Melatonin	3-15 mg daily, 8-12 p.m.	Circadian rhythm enhancement Sleep enhancement Neuroendocrine regulation	Arendt, et al., 1986 Dilman and Dean, 1992
Nimodipine	30 mg twice daily	Calcium-channel inhibition Vasodilation	see *SDII*: Nimodipine chapter
Phosphatidylserine	100 mg 3 times daily	Phospholipid nutrient support Membrane stabilization Methylation enhancement Membrane fluidization	see *SDII*: Phosphatidylserine chapter
Piracetam	800 mg 3 times daily	Cerebral metabolic enhancement	see *SDII*: Piracetam Update see *SD&N* references
Brewer's yeast /RNA	up to 15 grams as tolerated	Memory enhancement Nutritional support	Dalderup, et al., 1970 Munch-Petersen, et al., 1974

Possible Adjunctive Strategies

Substances	Dosages	Therapeutic effects	References
Krebs-cycle intermediates	As directed	Support of energy metabolism	Davies, 1981
Pyritinol	200 mg 3 times daily	Vasodilation Cerebral metabolic activation Cholinergic activation Cerebral circulation enhancement	Cooper and Magnus, 1980 Seyfried, 1989
AL 7:2:1 (egg-lipid preparation)	10 grams daily (up to 30 grams daily)	Membrane fluidization Membrane stabilization	Shinitzky, et al., 1983
L-Dopa	250-4,000 mg daily	Dopamine precursor loading	Kristensen, et al. 1977 Jellinger, et al., 1980

Treatment	Dosage	Mechanism	Reference
Tyrosine and phenylalanine	500-2000 mg in a.m.	Noradrenergic precursor loading	Gelenberg, et al., 1980
Bromocriptine	1.25-2.5 mg daily	Dopamine receptor stimulation / Prolactin suppression	Phuapradit, et al., 1978
Ondansetron	0.25-1.0 mg 2 times daily	Serotonin re-uptake inhibition (of 5-HT3 receptors)	see Ondansetron chapter references
L-Tryptophan	500-2000 mg before sleep	Serotonin precursor loading	Smith, Stromgren, et al., 1984
Cylert (pemoline)	18-75 mg daily	Psychostimulation	Bartus, 1979 / Ferris, 1981
TRH	as prescribed	Neuropeptide stimulation	Hollister, 1986
Thyroid hormone	0.25-0.5 mg daily	Hormone replacement therapy	Barnes and Galton, 1976
Chelation therapy	as administered	Heavy-metal elimination / Removal of aluminum and calcium cross-links	Cranton, 1992
Gangliosides	as prescribed	miscellaneous	
Hyperbaric oxygen	as administered	Improved oxygenation / Metabolic enhancement	Raskin, et al., 1978
or Oxygen (normobaric)	as administered or directed	Improved oxygenation / Metabolic enhancement	Jacobs, et al., 1969
or H_2O_2 (intravenous)	as administered	Improved oxygenation / Metabolic enhancement	Roberts, 1981
Trental	as prescribed	Increase RBC elasticity	Harwart, 1979
Tacrine (THA, Cognex)	25-200 mg, maximum tolerated dose	Cholinergic enhancement / Acetylcholinesterase inhibition	Farlo, 1992 / Molloy, 1991

Adapted and extensively revised from Bagne, et al., 1986.

approach should 1) be directed against the potential causes of the disease, 2) correct the deficiencies, 3) alleviate symptoms, and 4) provide general neuronal support. We developed our suggested therapeutic protocol by combining a number of individual therapeutic approaches, adapted from an outline originally presented by Bagne and colleagues [1986], which we have greatly modified, augmented, and updated (Table 1). The broad-spectrum multi-drug approach to Alzheimer's disease that we recommend uses four criteria for inclusion of any substance: 1) effectiveness, 2) availability, 3) cost, and 4) absence of toxicity.

Our suggested combined approach attacks Alzheimer's disease from many different directions, with very little overlap of mechanism for each component. Thus, nearly all bases are covered, with very little risk of adverse effects, and no known adverse cross-reaction between any of the substances listed. This combined approach is, however, experimental, and should not be under- taken without a physician's supervision. With the insidious, progressive downward course of Alzheimer's disease, the risk (compared to doing nothing) is certainly minimal, and the potential for dramatic improvement is substantial.

Therapeutic modalities should be tailored to the needs of the individual and the stage of the disease. The use of alcohol, tobacco and caffeine-containing beverages should be minimized. Care should be taken not to withdraw these items too rapidly, to minimize the stress of this process [Roberts, 1981].

A number of nutrients have been tested alone and in conjunction with other nutrients and drugs for Alzheimer's disease, with varying degrees of success (see references in Table 1). Our combined recommended protocol incorporates all nutrients that have either 1) demonstrated efficacy in clinical tests, or 2) a strong theoretical basis for potential benefit in Alzheimer's disease, even though they may not have been effective when tested as isolated nutrients. These substances are inexpensive, extremely safe, and may be of benefit by themselves — or they may augment other, more effective therapies. Inclusion of these nutrients appears to be in accord with Drachman and Glosser's recommendation [1981] to provide general metabolic support of neural function when developing treatment strategies.

Although this may at first appear to be quite a "drug and nutrient cocktail," it is no more complicated than the nutritional regimens that many people follow each day. An Alzheimer's patient should not, of course, be expected to carry out this regimen without supervision. However, family members or care providers can certainly set up a routine that can be easily carried out. Because of the non-toxic and non-habit-forming nature of all of the above substances, missed doses or even moderate overdoses are not particularly harmful.

We also believe that every Alzheimer's patient should have a complete thyroid work-up, to rule out overt or sub-clinical hypothyroidism. Many of the symptoms of hypothyroidism mimic those of Alzheimer's disease, and traditional blood tests are now recognized to be inadequate for accurate diagnosis. Appropriate doses of thyroid hormone may produce dramatic alterations in energy levels, depression, and cognitive function. I [WD] prefer Armour Desiccated Thyroid.

Another medication which has unfortunately fallen into undeserved disrepute is Cylert (pemoline), a controlled drug which is a derivative of amphetamine. Cylert may dramatically improve the somnolence (daytime sleepiness) of many Alzheimer's patients, and may also improve cognitive performance.

What About Tacrine (THA)?

Although tacrine (THA) has been recently recommended for FDA approval for use in treating Alzheimer's disease, we do not believe that it is more effective by itself than many other substances discussed in this book and in our previous book, *Smart Drugs & Nutrients*. In addition, in contrast to most of the substances that we have reviewed, tacrine (trade name Cognex) is fairly toxic, and its adverse effects may outweigh the modest benefits which may be obtained. This toxicity may prohibit many patients from taking it. This is definitely a subject which should be addressed by a physician.

Chelation Therapy

Chelation therapy is a treatment administered by physician members of the American College of Advancement in Medicine (for the name of an ACAM physician in your area, call 714-583-7666). It consists of multiple intravenous infusions of EDTA (ethylenediaminetetraacetic acid), a synthetic amino acid, in combination with selected vitamins and minerals.

Chelation therapy is used to treat a number of chronic degenerative conditions, including angina pectoris, intermittent claudication (reduced circulation in the muscles), coronary artery disease, diabetes, hypertension, and Alzheimer's disease. These treatments are usually administered once or twice a week, requiring about three hours per treatment. They are relatively painless and non-invasive (requiring only insertion of an IV needle), and usually administered in a pleasant social environment with other patients.

Chelation therapy is the most effective way to remove aluminum, a component of the neurofibrillary tangles found in the brains of Alzheimer's patients. I [WD] recommend a minimum course of twenty to thirty treatments be administered as early as possible in every Alzheimer's patient. For more information about chelation therapy, see Dr. Elmer Cranton's book, *Bypassing Bypass*, available from Medex Publishers, Inc. at 800-426-3551.

How Long Does it Take for Improvements to Occur?

Although some Alzheimer's patients show almost immediate improvement, many do not begin to improve for a minimum of six months. As an example, in a double-blind, placebo-controlled study of Hydergine on Alzheimer's disease patients,

Kugler and colleagues [1978] found no benefit from 6 months of Hydergine therapy. However, at a second follow-up 9 months later (15 months after the beginning of therapy), they found that the Hydergine group had improved 5-7% on the Wechsler Intelligence Test. Hoffer [1993] reports that one of his patients was worse after six months on a combined nutritional/aspirin therapy, but improved after ten months. Hoffer's patient continued to improve during two years of follow-up. These examples confirm that it is necessary to use prolonged therapy on Alzheimer's disease patients.

Since Alzheimer's disease is a chronic condition of many years duration, it will probably require an extended period of time for any truly significant therapeutic agent to alter its course. Physicians and researchers (and patients and family) must adopt an therapeutic attitude much like that which currently exists for cancer (i.e., five-year outcome).

For example, oncologists (cancer doctors) accept heroic measures including major surgery, whole-body irradiation, and chemotherapy in return for increases in five-year survival rates of 10% or less. However, just the opposite attitude prevails with respect to Alzheimer's disease. Everyone wants a short-term cure. If an agent does not exert a dramatic clinical effect in a short-term study, it is regarded as virtually useless by the research community. This attitude must change [Reisberg, 1981].

References

Altman H, Mehta D, Evenson RC, and Sletten IW. Behavioral effects of drug therapy on psychogeriatric inpatients. II. Multivitamin supplement???. *Journal of the American Geriatrics Society* 21: 249-52, 1973.

Bagne CA, Pomara N, Crook T, and Gershon S. Alzheimer's disease strategies for treatment and research. In: *Treatment Development Strategies for Alzheimer's Disease*, p. 585-638, Mark Powley Associates, Inc, New Canaan, 1986.

Barnes B, and Galton L. *Hypothyroidism — The Unsuspected Illness*. Harper and Row, New York, 1976.

Bartus RT. Four stimulants of the central nervous system: Effects on short-term memory in young versus aged monkeys. *J Am Geriatrics Soc* 27: 289-98, 1979.

Bowen DM, and Davison AM. Can the pathophysiology of dementia lead to rational therapy? In: *Treatment Development Strategies for Alzheimer's Disease*, p. 25-66, Mark Powley Associates, Inc, New Canaan, 1986.

Carlsson A. Aging and brain neurotransmitters. In: *Strategies for the Development of an Effective Treatment for Senile Dementia*, by Thomas Crook and Samuel Gershon (eds), p. 93-104, Mark Powley Associates, Inc., New Canaan, 1981.

Cherkin A. Effects of nutritional factors on memory function, In: *Nutritional Intervention in the Aging Process*, by H. James Armbrecht, John M. Predergast, and Rodney M. Coe (Eds.), p. 229-249, Springer-Verlag, New York, 1984.

Cohen GD. Senile Dementia of the Alzheimer Type (SDAT): Nature of the disorder, in: Strategies for the Development of an Effective Treatment for Senile Dementia, by Thomas Crook and Samuel Gershon (eds), 1981, Mark Powley Associates, Inc., New Canaan, 1-5.

Constantinidis J. The zinc-deficiency theory for the pathogenesis of neurofibrillary tangles: Possibility of preventive treatment by a zinc compound. *Neurobiology of Aging* 11: 282, 1990.

Constantinidis J. Treatment of Alzheimer's disease by zinc compounds. *Drug Development Research* 27: 1-14, 1992.

Cooper AJ, and Magnus RV. A placebo-controlled study of pyritinol ("Encephabol") in dementia. *Pharmacotherapeutica* 2: 317-322, 1980.

Cranton E. *Bypassing Bypass*. Medex Publishers, Ripshin Rd., 1992. (Medex Publishers, PO Box 44, Trout Dale, VA 24378-0044.

Czerwinski AW, Clark ML, Serafetinides EA, Perrier C, and Huber W. Safety and efficacy of zinc sulfate in geriatric patients. *Clinical Pharmacology and Therapeutics* 15: 436-41, 1974.

Dalderup LM, van Haard WB, Keller GHM, Dalmeier JF, Frijda NH, and Elshout JJ. An attempt to change memory and serum composition in old people by a daily supplement of dried baker's yeast. *J Gerontology* 25: 320-324, 1970.

Davies P. Theoretical treatment possiblilites for dementia of the Alzheimer Type: Cholinergic hypothesis. In: *Strategies for the Development of an Effective Treatment for Senile Dementia*, by Thomas Crook and Samuel Gershon (Eds), p. 19-32, Mark Powley Associates, Inc., New Canaan, 1981.

Deijen JB, van der Beek EJ, Orlebeke JF, and van den Berg H. Vitamin B-6 supplementation in elderly men: effects on mood, memory, performance and mental effort. *Psychopharmacology* 109: 489-496, 1992.

Drachman DA, and Glosser G. Pharmacologic strategies in aging and dementia: The cholinergic hypothesis. In: *Strategies for the Development of an Effective Treatment for Senile Dementia*, by Thomas Crook and Samuel Gershon (eds), p. 35-51, Mark Powley Associates, Inc., New Canaan, 1981.

Durso R, Fedio P, Brouwers P, Cox C, Martin AJ, Ruggieri SA, Tamminga CA, and Chase TN. Lysine vasopressin in Alzheimer's disease. *Neurology* 32: 674-77, 1982.

Etienne P. Treatment of Alzheimer's disease with lecithin. In: *Alzheimer's Disease*, by B. Reisberg (Ed), New York, Free Press, 1983.

Ferris SH. Empirical studies in senile dementia with central nervous system stimulants and metabolic enhancers. In: *Strategies for the Development of an Effective Treatment for Senile Dementia*, by Thomas Crook and Samuel Gershon (Eds), p. 173-187, Mark Powley Associates, Inc., New Canaan, 1981.

Fillit H, Weinreb H, Cholst I, Luine V, Amador R, Zabriskie JB, and McEwen BS. Hormonal therapy for Alzheimer's disease. In: *Treatment Development Strategies for Alzheimer's Disease*, Mark Powley Associates, Inc, New Canaan, 1986.

Fisman M, Mersky H, and Helmes E. Double-blind trial of 2-dimethylaminoethanol in Alzheimer's disease. *American Journal of Psychiatry* 138: 970-972, 1981.

Gibson GE, and Peterson C. Consideration of neurotransmitters and calcium metabolism in therapeutic design. In: *Treatment Development Strategies for*

Alzheimer's Disease, p. 499-517, Mark Powley Associates, Inc, New Canaan, 1986.

Glick JL. Dementias: The role of magnesium deficiency and an hypothesis concerning the pathogenesis of Alzheimer's disease. *Medical Hypotheses* 31: 211-25, 1990a.

Glick JL. Use of magnesium in the management of dementias. *Med Sci Res* 18: 831-33, 1990b.

Goldsmith MF. Youngest institute addresses aging problems. *JAMA* 252: 2315-17, 1984.

Gottfries CG. Etiological and treatment considerations in SDAT. In: *Strategies for the Development of an Effective Treatment for Senile Dementia*, by Thomas Crook and Samuel Gershon (Eds), p. 107-20, Mark Powley Associates, Inc., New Canaan, 1981.

Harwart D. The treatment of chronic cerebrovascular insufficiency. A double-blind study with pentoxifylline (Trental 400). *Current Medical Research and Opinion* 6: 73-84, 1979.

Hoffer A. A case of Alzheimer's treated with nutrients and aspirin. *J Orthomolecular Medicine* 8(1): 43-44, 1993.

Hollister L. An overview of strategies for the Development of an effective treatment for senile dementia. In: *Strategies for the Development of an Effective Treatment for Senile Dementia*, by Thomas Crook and Samuel Gershon (eds), p. 7-16, Mark Powley Associates, Inc., New Canaan, 1981.

Imagawa M. Megavitamin therapy (Coenzyme Q_{10} and Vitamin B_6) in Alzheimer's disease and SDAT. In: *Basic, Cliinical and Therapeutic Aspects of Alzheimer's and Parkinson's Diseases*, Volume 2, by T. Nagatsu, *et al.*, (Eds), p. 489-91, Plenum Press, New York, 1990.

Imagawa M, Naruse S, Tsuji S, Fujioka A, and Yamaguchi H. Coenzyme Q_{10}, iron and vitamin B_6 in genetically-confirmed Alzheimer's disease. *The Lancet* 340: 671, 1992.

Jacobs EA, Winter JPM, Alvis HJ, *et al.* Hyperoxygenation effects on cognitive functioning in the aged. *New Engl J Med* 281: 753, 1969.

Jellinger K, Flament H, Riederer P, Schmid H, and Ambrozi L. Levodopa in the treatment of presenile dementia. *Mechanisms of Ageing and Development* 14: 253-264, 1980.

Kral VA, Solyom L, Enesco H, and Ledwidge B. Relationship of vitamin B_{12} and folic acid to memory function. *Biological Psychiatry* 2: 19-26, 1970.

Kristensen V, Olsen M, and Theilgaard A. Levodopa treatment of presenile dementia. *Acta Psychiatrica Scandinavica* 55: 41-51, 1977.

Kruck TPA, Lukiw WJ, Serrao C, and McLachlan DRC. Molecular shuttle chelation — Studies on desferroxamine based chelation of aluminum for neurobiological applications: Alzheimer's Disease. *Neurobiology of Aging* 11: 342, 1990.

Kugler J, Oswald WD, Herzfeld U, *et al.* Langzeittherapie altersbedingter insuffizienzerscheinungen des Gehirns. *Deutsch Med Wochenschr* 103: 456-462, 1978.

LaBrecque DC, and Goldberg RI. A double-blind study of pentylenetetrazol combined with niacin in senile patients. *Current Therapeutic Research* 9: 611-617, 1967.

Laczi F, Zs V, Laszlo FA, Wagner A, Jardanhazy T, Szasz A, Szhard J, and Telegdy G. Effects of lysine-vasopressin and L-deamino-8-D-arginine-vasopressin on memory in healthy individuals and diabetes insipidus patients. *Psychoneuroendocrinology* 7: 185-89, 1982.

Landfield PW. Preventive approaches to normal brain aging and Alzheimer's disease. In: *Treatment Development Strategies for Alzheimer's Disease*, p. 221-43, Mark

Powley Associates, Inc, New Canaan, 1986.

Loriaux SM, Deijen JB, Orlebeke JF, and De Swart JH. The effects of nicotinic acid and xanthinol nicotinate on human memory in different categories of age — A double blind study. *Psychopharmacology* 87: 390-95, 1985.

Lyte M, and Shinitzky M. Possible reversal of tissue aging by a lipid diet. In: *Alzheimer's disease: Advances in basic research and therapies*, RJ Wurtman, SH Corkin, and JH Growdon (Eds), p. 295-312, Center for Brain Sciences and Metabolism Charitable Trust, Zurich, 1983.

McDonald RJ. Hydergine: A review of 26 clinical studies. *Pharmakopsychiatrie* 12: 407-422, 1979.

McGeer PL, McGeer EG, Rogers J, and Sibley J. Does anti-inflammatory treatment protect against Alzheimer's disease? In: *Alzheimer's Disease — New Treatment Strategies*, by Zaven S. Khachaturian, and John Blass (Eds), p. 165-171, Marcel Dekker, Inc., New York, 1993.

Munch-Peterson S, Pakkenberg H, Kornerup H, Ortmann J, Ipsen E, Jacobsen P, and Simmel-Sgard H. RNA treatment of dementia. *Acta Neurologica Scandinavica* 50: 553-72, 1974.

Nandy K. Lipofuscin pigment and immunological factors in the pathogenesis and treatment of senile dementia. In: *Strategies for the Development of an Effective Treatment for Senile Dementia*, by Thomas Crook and Samuel Gershon (Eds), p. 231-45, Mark Powley Associates, Inc., New Canaan, 1981.

Parker LN, Levin ER, and Lifrak ET. Evidence for adrenocortical adaptation to severe illness. *J Clinical Endocrinology and Metabolism* 60: 947-953, 1985.

Phuapradit P, Phillips M, Lees AJ, and Stern GM. Bromocriptine in presenile dementia. *British Medical Journal* 1: 1052-53, 1978.

Raskin AS, Gershon S, Crook T, Sathananthan G, and Ferns S. The effects of hyperbaric and normobaric oxygen on cognitive impairment in the elderly. *Archives of General Psychiatry* 139: 1468-71, 1978.

Reisberg B. Empirical studies in senile dementia with metabolic enhancers and agents that alter blood flow and oxygen utilization. In: *Strategies for the Development of an Effective Treatment for Senile Dementia*, by Thomas Crook and Samuel Gershon (Eds), p. 189-206, Mark Powley Associates, Inc., New Canaan, 1981.

Roberts E. Potential therapies in aging and senile dementias. *Annals of the New York Academy of Sciences* 396: 165-78, 1982.

Roberts E. A speculative consideration of the neurobiology and treatment of senile dementia. In: *Strategies for the Development of an Effective Treatment for Senile Dementia*, by Thomas Crook and Samuel Gershon (Eds), p. 247-320, Mark Powley Associates, Inc., New Canaan, 1981.

Roberts E. Guides through the labyrinth of AD: Dehydroepiandrosterone, potassium channels, and the C4 component of complement. In: *Treatment Development Strategies for Alzheimer's Disease*, 173-219, Mark Powley Associates, Inc, New Canaan, 1986.

Rotrosen John. Membrane lipids: Can modification reduce symptoms or halt progression in Alzheimer's disease? In: *Treatment Development Strategies for Alzheimer's Disease*, 519-37, Mark Powley Associates, Inc, New Canaan, 1986.

Sapolsky RM, and McEwan BS. Stress, glucocorticoids, and their role in the aging hippocampus. In: *Treatment Development Strategies for Alzheimer's Disease*, 151-71, Mark Powley Associates, Inc, New Canaan, 1986.

Seyfried CA. Neurochemical effects of pyritinol and their relevance for the treatment of brain function deficits in old age. *Drug Development Research* 18: 1-9, 1989.

Shaw DM, MacSweeney DA, Johnson AL, O'Keefe R, Naidoo D, Macleod DM, Jog S,

Preece JM, and Crowley JM. Folate and amine metabolites in senile dementia: A combined trial and biochemical study. *Psychological Medicine* 1: 166-171, 1971.

Smith DF, Stromgren E, Petersen HN, Williams DG, and Sheldon W. Lack of effect of tryptophan treatment in demented gerontopsychiatric patients. *Acta Psychiatrica Scandinavica* 70: 470-477, 1984.

Thal LJ, Rosen W, Sharpless NS, and Crystal H. Choline chloride fails to improve cognition in Alzheimer's disease. *Neurobiology of Aging* 2: 205-8, 1981.

U. S. Department of Health and Human Services. Alzheimer's disease: Report of the Secretary's Task Force on Alzheimer's Disease (DHHS Publication No. [ADM] 84-1323). Washington, D.C., U.S. Government Printing Office.

Weiner MA. *Reducing the Risk of Alzheimer's*, Briarcliff Manor, Stein and Day, 1987.

Weingartner H, Kaye W, Gold P, Smallberg S, Peterson R, Gillin JC, and Ebert M. Vasopressin treatment of cognitive dysfunction in progressive dementia. *Life Sciences* 29: 2721-26, 1981.

Whitman RM. Re-evaluation of a glutamate-vitamin-iron preparation (L-glutavite) in the treatment of geriatric chronic brain syndrome with special reference to research design. *Journal of the American Geriatrics Society* 24: 859-870, 1966.

Suggested Treatment Protocol

Part II:

People of the Smart Drug Revolution

Part II: People of the Smart Drug Revolution

Smart Drug Users

We have received hundreds of stories from smart drug users since the publication of *Smart Drugs & Nutrients*. We have tried to include here a selection of these personal accounts, positive and negative, representing a wide cross-section of people, lifestyles, and personalities: a computer programmer able to "hold more code" in his head, a woman now able to remember the long numbers required of her in her job, a student with increased sex drive, an airline pilot using piracetam because his passengers are "safer" when he uses it, an elderly bridge player whose bridge scores improved, an artist who claims, "I've got my future back!" and more. A picture will begin to emerge of the 'smart drug scene' as just plain folks improving their performance in small but significant ways.

But note that these stories do not constitute any sort of proof in the scientific sense. The smart drug sections in other parts of this book are all based on scientific studies, described in mainstream professional scientific journals. Many of the studies are double-blind, placebo-controlled studies which clearly document the efficacy of smart drugs on normal, healthy humans, aging humans, or people with Alzheimer's disease.

Some scientists have criticized our inclusion of people's personal smart drug stories as being anecdotal and irrelevant. If these testimonials were the only substantiation of our premise, we would agree. However, we suggest that researchers read this section carefully and with an open mind. Important research always starts with observation. Only through observation can a researcher decide what theory to test. There are many wonderful and useful observations in this section, and some even suggest ideas for fascinating scientific studies, as you will read.

Please send us your stories for inclusion in *Smart Drugs III*! See the tearout card in the front of this book for details.

An Airline Pilot's Experience

"As a pilot for a major airline, I looked into the use of cognitive enhancers in an effort to optimize my performance. I have been using piracetam for a year and have noted a marked improvement in my abilities to keep track of all details involved in flying a large airliner.

"The sheer amount of data that a pilot must keep track of is sometimes overwhelming. With the use of Piracetam, I feel that I am better suited to take stock of issues such as the position of other planes, changing flight instructions and conflicting information regarding landing and flight plans which are apt to change at a moment's notice.

"Over all, I think that my passengers and crew are in safer hands when I am using piracetam, and I plan to continue its use as a personal edge in my work.

"Please don't give out my name because if my employers heard of my use of piracetam I could lose my job."

Anonymous airline pilot
Dallas, Texas

A Journalist's Story

Jeff Greenwald, a freelance writer, is one of the few journalists covering smart drugs to publicly admit to experimenting with them. In his front page article (December 22, 1991) in the *LA Times Magazine* he describes an informal, but very interesting, experiment he conducted: he had an educational psychologist test his IQ before and after using a mix of smart drugs.

Mr. Greenwald took daily doses of Hydergine, piracetam, and Choline Cooler™ (a smart drink designed by life extension authors/scientists Durk Pearson and Sandy Shaw). These drugs were described in our earlier book, *Smart Drugs & Nutrients*.

Greenwald's IQ was tested by Dr. Greg Larson (an expert in this area). Greenwald scored significantly higher on the second test, only four weeks after starting his smart drug program. The most dramatic improvements, according to Larson, were in the areas of short-term memory and sustained concentration.

In Greenwald's article he describes his subjective experiences several weeks into the experiment:

"I began to notice — or thought I noticed — some subtle but unmistakable changes. To begin with, I found that I was speaking more fluently. At 37, I sometimes get stalled in mid-sentence, unable to find the specific word I'm looking for. But suddenly, I was able to recall words at will. And not just words; telephone numbers, names, movie schedules, shopping lists and other bits of informational effluvia also seemed to spend more time in my short-term memory.

"These changes, admittedly, were subtle. Maybe they were the result of the intense focus and concentration I had to muster in order to write about neuroscience in the first place. Nor was I liberated from memory lapses completely; I still wandered into rooms on errands, the nature of which slipped my mind the moment I arrived. Once, I folded up a blanket and absent-mindedly walked into the kitchen to put it in the oven.

"In addition to the apparent memory enhancement, the drugs had another salubrious effect, which I almost hesitate to report. Impossible as it is to qualify, I found that my intuition — the part of my psyche that anticipates things or guesses other people's thoughts — was sharper. Time and again I guessed, accurately, what a friend was thinking, or what someone was about to say.

"Do I consider any of this scientific evidence? Not at all. But if I wanted to believe it, there it was."

A Movie Producer's Experience

"I'm a writer/director/producer with credits in film, television, theater and even music. I have taken Hydergine since the early 80s, after reading about it in Durk Pearson and Sandy Shaw's Life Extension. *But John Morgenthaler's articles and Morgenthaler's and Dean's original book,* Smart Drugs & Nutrients, *got me experimenting with smart drugs in earnest.*

"Daily, I take Hydergine, piracetam, choline, phosphatidylserine and Ginkgo biloba. *When I'm working, and especially when I'm working under pressure, I might use Diapid for concentrating, and centrophenoxine, sulbutiamine and/or vinpocetine for recall. Each of these drugs, individually and in combination, has increased my mental clarity and stamina. But the most amazing improvement has been in my work.*

"Writer's block is now a thing of the past. I am quicker and more articulate with my thoughts, not just on paper, but in public as well, whether at parties or at meetings to pitch new projects.

"I just finished a two-year stint on the science fiction series, Super Force. *I was supervising producer the first season, and in two seasons my partners and I wrote 35 episodes! Twenty of those episodes were written in an amazing 14-week sprint! The show had good ratings and won several awards. Three of our scripts came in first, second and third place for the Crystal Reel Award given by the Florida Film Commission.*

"As a writer/producer in episodic television, you're really working simultaneously on half-a-dozen episodes or more. You're preparing a story to pitch to the production company, you're writing the episode they've just approved, you're rewriting and prepping an episode that's about to shoot, you're overseeing and rewriting the episode that's shooting, you're reworking and supervising the episode that was just shot and is now being edited, and you're writing new lines for and making the final adjustments to the episode that's ready to go out. As you sit down for a rest, an actor may walk up to you and ask 'Why do I say this?' You've got to know what script he's talking about and have a reasonable answer even if you wrote the line five weeks ago. I've never had a problem since taking smart drugs.

"And it's not just for work. I seem to be at peak efficiency constantly. That helps in a business where being in the right place at the right time and saying the right thing is important. Forearmed is forearmed."

Jeff Mandel
Los Angeles, California

Comment: Jeff is modest. He's also written for the CBS sci-fi series *Otherworld*, and was Executive Script Consultant on ABC's *O'Hara*. He has directed several science fiction, action and horror films including *Elves, Robo-C.H.I.C.* (which he also wrote), and *Firehead* starring Christopher Plummer and Martin Landau (which he wrote). He was head writer for and directed National Lampoon's review *Sex, Drugs, Rock & Roll, And The End Of The World*, and he wrote *Teen Wolf III* which begins shooting in Fall '93. Mr. Mandel is also a composer of music for films and television, and recently produced an album for the up-and-coming pop star, Steen.

Jeff has been a good friend, and also a tireless speaker-to-journalists-about-smart-drugs. All of us appreciate him and the dozens of other people willing to put their reputations on the line in front of the TV cameras or journalists' tape decks.

A Bridge Player

"I am the 'elderly bridge player' who appeared on the Dateline *program aired by NBC on June 2, 1992. There were several significant errors, omissions, and misquotes in my short appearance.*

"My bridge game actually deteriorated 15 years ago (not last year, as they stated on the show). I did not say I was winning all the time, now. Instead, I gave them, in writing (from my computer) statistical data proving the improvement after taking the drugs. The crew ignored what I told them during the eight hours they were here.

"In Dateline's *interviews with the medical 'authorities,' it was implied that all smart drug users experiment on their own. I have been under an M.D.'s close supervision. The medical authorities were never told that I had given NBC cold statistics showing improvement using the prescriptions. NBC seemed to agree that all improvements were subjective, and that a scientific study was impossible, as there was no mathematical way that performance could be measured and compared.*

"Duplicate bridge would be ideal for such a study for the following four reasons:

1. *There is a national organization in which bridge players are members. Each member has a membership number which could be used for identification of the volunteers for the study.*

2. *The organization, The American Contract Bridge League [ACBL], sets rules and supervises several thousand bridge clubs. They provide a computer program that is the same for every club, so that all results are valid for comparison. They have national ratings of their members the same way the PGA ranks golfers and the Tennis Association ranks tennis players.*

3. *There is a computer record of every club game played. The most meaningful figure on this record is the figure known as 'percentage of game.'*

4. *Bridge requires excellent concentration and short-term memory. Competition is fierce. Over half of the members are seniors over the age of 55. Most play an average of three games a week.*

"In my case, my percentage of game was 42% in the year prior to starting smart drugs. Since taking the drugs, my percentage has risen to an average of 55%. A professional expert in the ACBL will perform at an average of 60% when playing in games open to all members (not when playing in games open to experts only)."

Paul Chalfant
Colton, California

Comment: We are not surprised that *Dateline* chose to gloss over the scientific and medical aspects of Paul's story (Remember, this is the same show which fraudulently blew up a General Motors truck). In 1991 and 1992, journalists chose the question, "Do smart drugs work?" as the point on which to balance their stories. Already, we've noticed a trend to, "Should people have access to smart drugs?" as the balancing point. We think that Paul's happiness, satisfaction and productivity speak to that issue more effectively than anything we could say.

A Family's Experience

"Our first experience with smart drugs was in using piracetam with DMAE. We were hoping to improve our memory, but were delighted with the mood improvement, the feeling of being in control, and extra energy. We used both DMAE and piracetam alone and found neither gave us the same effect when used by themselves.

"After adding Hydergine in a very small amount, and later deprenyl, I feel that I have my memory back as it was when I was much younger. I have a built-in test in my work to gauge memory improvement. Working with jobs at a computer, I must repeatedly during the day consult an old job for disc number (four to five digits) and job number (another four or five digits). Before taking smart drugs I found myself constantly having to refer back to the old job after locating the proper floppy disc, because I had by that time forgotten the job number. Every day now, I am delighted that I no longer have to do this. I had been having trouble remembering complete phone numbers with area codes long enough to walk from the rolodex to the fax machine and dial the complete number. Now I have no problem with this, either. The wonderful antidepressant effect has come as a bonus.

"A quote from my daughter, who is 34 and has also been taking piracetam, DMAE and deprenyl: 'I feel like I must have had a deprenyl deficiency all my life. Now I have energy and ambition. I feel like I've always thought other people must feel.' She takes the low dosage recommended by you in Smart Drug News.

"My husband is an artist who has, since the age of thirty, bemoaned the fact that he was not already famous, and felt that he was too old to be successful. Now, he says 'I've got my future back.'

"Since we've started on this regimen, his output has increased tremendously. He has more ideas than he has time to execute. He has taken the initiative to sell his work in more outlets and has had success with this. Instead of feeling like his life is over, he feels like there is much more to be done. The piracetam and DMAE

in particular have helped for nervousness when making speeches, which he has had to do at show openings.

"Thanks very much to Dean and Fowkes for answers to several of my questions in the last issue of the newsletter. I appreciate it.

"Last week I had the first letter from the FDA on a package seizure. Between us, my daughter and I have probably ordered 40 or 50 packages. I immediately sent a prescription to the FDA in Baltimore, and today received the release form, so I assume I will be getting the package soon. It is piracetam from Mougios in Greece.

"Keep up the good work. We need you!"

JC
Benton, Arkansas

Chronic Fatigue & Nootropics

"It was quite by chance that I saw a Donahue show about SD&N *in December, 1991, I believe. That show opened some important doors. After reading through your book, and getting order forms from one of the overseas suppliers, I placed an order for phenytoin, piracetam, and vasopressin. The order took about six weeks to arrive.*

"My interest in nootropics comes from suffering with chronic fatigue syndrome (CFS). As a result of your show I asked my CFS specialist if I could try Hydergine, which he prescribed. I began taking the phenytoin, piracetam, and vasopressin in small amounts, and found after about four days I was feeling too energetic, even manic. That was not the result I wanted, so I cut back to just phenytoin. The results I had were similar to what Jack Dreyfus described in his book, A Remarkable Medicine Has Been Overlooked. *My insomnia went away and more energy appeared.*

"I have been using Piracetam in place of caffeine and Vasopressin when I become very lethargic. For me, CFS has a cycling affect. When more ill with CFS I am more lethargic and fatigued. There are other symptoms as well but, lethargy, fatigue, and memory problems are the most common and troubling. When less ill with CFS there is less lethargy and less need for stimulants.

"My wife and I have spent a lot of money and time trying to find out what I had in the first place. Evidently, I contracted CFS about 23 years ago. In October 1991, I received a diagnosis of CFS.

"We took a chance in ordering those three medications, since there was no promise that they would work, but they did! I am so grateful you have put together the book, SD&N. *I am part of a CFS Support Group, and recently spoke for over an hour to them about your book and the medications I have tried. Many were very interested.*

"As I told them, I still have CFS, but there are other medications that may help alleviate some of the serious effects of CFS, like missing our memories, and this constant state of fatigue and lethargy.

"I was glad to discover caffeine, seven years after getting CFS. However, caffeine only got me close to feeling normal. Sometimes, it did not work at any dosage. Phenytoin, piracetam, and vasopressin have changed that. I feel more normal, not excitable or nervous, as when I was on caffeine.

"Gentlemen, you have opened many doors for me and many others who suffer the effects of Chronic Fatigue Syndrome (or CFIDS, Chronic Fatigue Immune Deficiency Syndrome)."

SGD
Sacramento, California

Smart Drugs and Alcoholism

"I have had a knowledge of health foods and natural healing since about 1969. I have been continually learning since then, and practicing eating fruit, veggies, vitamins, supplements, fasting and also experimenting with drugs, some of which I have found to be destructive.

"Recently, however, I saw you on TV and read your book. I have been trying piracetam, choline, B_5 and Hydergine for a couple of weeks. The piracetam totally cured me of alcohol addiction. I can't stand the sight of it (alcohol) anymore, and haven't had a drop for seven days. I am sure you're onto something big here,

and I encourage you to continue with wisdom and discretion. I am taking 800 mg piracetam with three grams choline, 450 mg B5, and 1.5 mg Hydergine per day. I felt very helped by this combination after only two days. Keep up the good work."

RM
Mexico

Comment: Thank you for your story. Please stay in touch — we would like to hear what happens.

Dilantin and Obsession

"I had already been taking a high-potency vitamin/antioxidant formula a few times daily for a long time when I decided to try DMAE. After several days, I built up to three to five 350 mg tablets daily. I found that it definitely increased my mental alertness and my physical energy. I would not call the effects truly stimulatory, rather, I just felt better. It took a couple of weeks to really notice a difference.

"I decided to order some piracetam from an overseas mail-order firm several weeks after beginning the DMAE. I did not notice any difference at all for several days. Then, suddenly, I felt the difference strongly. My ability to see connections between and within ideas, my verbal ability, and my powers of concentration have all markedly increased. As a student, I find piracetam (2400 mg daily) truly helpful.

"Then I got curious about Dilantin. I'd read bits and snatches about this medication in many publications, but I was most interested in the possibility of it helping me with a mild but persistent problem with compulsive eating. Although it had been tried on bulemics with mixed results, I thought that compulsive eating and bulemia might be related, and decided to try it anyway. I picked a low dose (25 mg three times daily) because of my concerns about toxicity.

"I did not expect results, yet the food obsession disappeared. I used to think about food all day, making calorie/nutrient lists, making eating plans, and more. I am now 33 years old and have been a compulsive eater and food obsessor since I was 12! It has

freed up a lot of my mental energy formerly wasted worrying about grams of fat and number of calories!

"I have also received good results with dimethylglycine (DMG). It's a mild euphoriant, helps me wake up on mornings after a rough night, increases my sex drive, and seems to increase my physical stamina. Like DMAE, DMG doesn't make me high, just well. I do not use it every day, I save it for occasions when I'd otherwise be tired or burned out.

"I'd like to try Hydergine next, but the FDA has threatened the companies from which I can buy it. I consider myself a careful and informed consumer and I very strongly resent the FDA playing Daddy. I prefer to make my own health choices."

SM

"I am a 37 year-old man. I take deprenyl, although I have never noticed any effects from it whatsoever. I take it on faith, because the research I've seen about its life-extending effects look so convincing."

JW
San Francisco, California

A Changed Person

"I have been giving my mother piracetam, centrophenoxine (Lucidril), and choline for a number of years. She is 84 years old with senile dementia. Before the introduction of these smart drugs, she had suffered strokes which left her terribly agitated. She would scream and holler uncontrollably.

"After smart drugs, she was a totally different person. Her agitation vanished, she stopped screaming and hollering, and her IQ went up tremendously. She can now hold intelligent conversations.

"Don't let anyone tell you that smart drugs don't work. I have living proof with my dear mother. I myself use some of the smart drugs. It's too bad the American public doesn't realize that without the FDA's restrictions, these wonderful medicines would be available for their benefit. Very sad."

RO

Comment: These observations, while anecdotal, are encouraging and serve to illustrate that smart drugs can't be easily dismissed as useless. It is interesting that the pharmaceutical company Warner-Lambert is conducting studies of piracetam for the treatment of Alzheimer's disease. Hopefully, this research will confirm this person's observations.

"I've been using DMAE-H3, manufactured by Twinlab, for six months and have been very pleased with the results. I noticed a significant increase in my attention span. This allows me to read for longer periods of time and retain more information.

"I've added Ginkgo biloba *extract (Solaray), ephedra (Solaray), and Super Strength Lecithin Phosphatidyl Choline Complex with B12, folic acid and linoleic acid (Nature's Plus) to my daily dosage of DMAE-H3 with no results.*

"I believe I've reached a plateau with DMAE-H3 and am seeking greater results, which I hope to achieve by adding aniracetam and Hydergine to my daily regimen. I hope I can successfully mail order these drugs.

"Thank you for writing the book and providing a means by which I can excel to new heights unattainable before your publication."

AW
Las Vegas, Nevada

"Chinese herbs (ephedra, schizandra), amino acids, and vitamins allow more rapid communication between both brain hemispheres. I used to consume piracetam and deprenyl until the FDA stopped my supply. These chemicals do work!"

SP
Mequon, Wisconsin

"I have used Deanol, ginseng, Ginkgo biloba, *Brain Pep and phenylalanine. It seems that at times I will have negative results.*

I've noticed that the more phenylalanine I take, the quicker my verbal responses are to any given situation."

SF
New Hope, Pennsylvania

"I've been using DMAE, choline, ginkgo (250 mg), ginseng (Korean), and Royal Jelly for five months. I have noticed an improvement in short-term and long-term memory. Also, my friends have noticed an improvement in my general disposition."

BB
Indian Rocks Beach, Florida

"DMAE has produced mild anxiety at high dosages when taken too soon in a program. Ginseng has proven to be strangely energetic and calming at the same time. L-Tyrosine has produced emotionally calming effects stopping short of actually enhancing a positive mood. DMAE has also, in lower dosages, enhanced planning and decision-making abilities. B-complex vitamins are excellent for general stamina and energy increase."

JS
Columbus, Ohio

Recovering from an Automobile Accident

"I have an incredible story to relate to you concerning smart drugs and nutrients. It is 100% true with no false statements. It would please me to see it in Volume II of your book as I hope it may help others.

"I am currently a 36 year old male, and am a Ph.D. student in environmental engineering at Southern Illinois University. I have a M.S. in biochemistry and have used neuroactive agents to enhance memory and cognition for many years. Unfortunately, in October of 1990 I was involved in a head-on auto accident and I was not buckled up. I suffered a terrible head injury and had what is termed a traumatic brain injury (TBI). I underwent neurosurgery for evacuation of four subdural hygromas. Neuro-logically, my deficits were quantified approximately 2 ½ months

post-TBI in a neuropsychological exam I undertook at a traumatic brain injury rehabilitation hospital. It showed a markedly diminished cognitive ability, as my IQ was in the mentally retarded range (68). Further, my short-term memory was completely gone as I literally could not remember anything for longer than a few seconds. The doctor told my family that only 3% of people with such injuries ever work again, even at the most menial tasks, and only about 1% ever fully regain their pre-injury intellect. Of course, I was unable to help myself as I could remember nothing about smart drugs and nutrients — or anything else. Well, things began to change about five months post-TBI. A friend, whom I previously turned on to the effects of smart drugs and nutrients some years earlier, provided me with a large amount of choline and pantothenic acid. I was given the supplied material to take several times per day (in retrospect I was taking about 5000 mg/day.) Well, over the next few weeks I started to slowly come around. As time went on — and I continued taking these neuroactive nutrients — I steadily improved, and at 13 months post-TBI I was discharged from the rehabilitation hospital and I shortly began work as an environmental engineer! It is now 2½ years post-TBI and I am working on my engineering Ph.D.!

"And to think I would have spent the rest of my life in that hospital had I not taken these marvelous, cheap, safe, and extremely effective nutrients. In fact, the hospital neuropsychologist told me I've made the best recovery he has ever seen.

"In conclusion, John, I will be happy to provide the name and address of the hospital, my doctor, or further elaboration; just call or write."

JFT
Carbondale, Illinois

"I have an attention deficit disorder for which most (all) physicians prescribe Ritalin (a cleaned street drug, by my

standards). I have been using piracetam, and it works 100% better. Thank you for making this book."

RD
Fort Wayne, Indiana

"Every time I had to take exams my pulse was skyrocketing! As a result, I couldn't concentrate and do my best. Thanks to Inderal, all this has stopped."

AR
Thessaloniki, Greece

"I have been taking a combination of Ginkgo, DMAE (my husband buys it for me in the States), choline bitartrate, glutamine, vitamins and minerals all this year. My low-level depression/mood swings are down, and my drive and creativity are up.

"I initiated a double-blind study on low-level and rheumatoid arthritis, which I presented in London at an international conference this year. This would have been impossible without the help of the above-mentioned substances.

"I just ordered Hydergine and piracetam as well as some Inderal for my brother-in-law. Will keep you posted. I am a physio-therapist working in a major teaching hospital in Sydney, but have been unable to find an interested physician to work with."

GH
Sydney, Australia

"I used Hydergine while learning Spanish. I was living in Colombia, S.A., and became fluent in eight months. I feel the use of it was the key."

NPT
Ocala, Florida

"My experience with smart drugs is fascinating in that my mental, emotional, and spiritual perceptions are sharper, clearer, deeper. I'm sure drugs can be helpful in increasing ones's capacity to live fully and alertly and consciously."

JM
Syracuse, New York

"I am currently taking choline, DMAE, B5, CoQ10, and Ginkgo. Fantastic!"

WA
Santa Monica, California

The Professor and Piracetam

"My husband, who was 80 this September, began by taking Hydergine. I had been very careful of his diet and made sure that he had well above the RDA vitamin intake. My ideas of vitamin consumption came first from Adelle Davis, then Vitamin C and the Common Cold *came along, then* Life Extension, *and at long last, just when things were beginning to look fairly hopeless in the area of senility,* Smart Drugs & Nutrients *came along. My husband is now taking 4800 mg of piracetam a day and having no problems with it at all, and certainly his memory is on the mend, but you'll have to take my word for that. Of course, he is still teaching for the University of Middlesex here in England. That should tell you something. I would extend his intake, but it is rather expensive. Still, I am thinking of trying deprenyl and see how she goes.*

"Let me point out that my husband has not been on his own; I have tried all these things myself. At this writing, however, I find I have some few problems with the piracetam. I get sharp pains in my head and lesser pains in my heart. My doctor suggested that I give the piracetam a pass. I truly had no idea of its being a problem, but the pain is gone; that must mean something."

SWT
Bluntisham, England

Comment: Thank you for your story, your intelligence and your pluck, madam. We especially appreciate that you carefully evaluated piracetam for yourself and found that it was not for you. Due to biochemical individuality, one person's favorite smart drug is another's headache. Congratulations on your diligence, it has paid off. Please stay in touch: we are very curious at what age (if ever!) your husband will retire.

Smart Drugs and Stroke

"I suffered a stroke on February 13, 1991, and thought all hope was gone to have a meaningful recovery, until I found a copy of SD&N *in a local health food store in late January, 1992. After reading your book, I began a course of self-medication (because the doctors I was seeing were very skeptical of the value of the medications I was inquiring about). I started taking nine mg of Hydergine, 1600 mg of piracetam, 15 mg of vinpocetine, 400 mg of DMAE, 50 mg of KH3, 180 mg of* Ginkgo biloba, *and 3000 mg of phosphatidylcholine a day, supplemented with other vitamins and minerals.*

"I have been taking these medications for the last nine months, and although I can't say that I have had a complete recovery (I don't think that ever happens), I have seen remarkable results. I am back to work full-time, and even my skeptical doctors are impressed with the results."

HWG
Semmes, Alabama

Comment: It's not always easy doing what we do but letters like this one make it all worthwhile.

"A year ago, I started taking Memory Fuel from Pearson and Shaw three times a day after reading about it in Smart Drugs & Nutrients. *A week later, I already had more concentration and energy. After a month I added Personal Radical Shield, building up to four capsules per meal, and again I felt this boost of energy.*

Now, a year later, I am stronger and healthier than ever before and I have not had a cold or flu in a year."

RvT
Amsterdam, Netherlands

"I am currently taking 1000 mg DMAE per day and notice a real difference in my alertness, energy level and decreased need for sleep. I'm looking forward to trying it with piracetam and Hydergine."

RS
Seattle, Washington

"I've been taking DMAE for several weeks, and I've notice an amazing difference in mood and concentration level. I've yet to try other nutrients, no drugs yet."

AFB
Austin, Texas

"I've had lots of success with combinations of niacin, pyro-glutamate, and choline, affecting my memory and mental alertness. I would like to try piracetam. But I know someone who lost a lot of money. He sent an order to Mexico, but hasn't received the piracetam or his money back."

STS
Erial, New Jersey

Comment: We are sorry your friend lost money. Our news-letter, *Smart Drug News* dedicates a great deal of time and effort to confirming the reliability of sources for smart drugs. We hope to eventually initiate laboratory testing for drugs. To subscribe, fill out the tear-out card at the front of this book and mail it in.

"I started using a product called Mental Edge from Source Naturals. The results were inconclusive. Then, I found a

distributor of Durk Pearson and Sandy Shaw products. I started using Memory Fuel and Fast Blast. I have much more energy and enthusiasm. I have been losing excess fat. As far as mental functioning is concerned, I have more stamina, and I don't get mentally distressed during long periods of concentration. I seem to be able to remember more information at work. Some of the more obscure information I remember doesn't have a context. Example, I may remember a name I saw once on a piece of paper, but I won't remember where or when."

KBS
Blaine, Minnesota

"Just started two months ago taking Mental Edge by Source Naturals. Also, L-Carnitine by NOW, choline, lecithin and vitamin E. All due to the Omni article that cited your book. My chess game has improved, but there are too many variables to be certain of improvement. Looking to add vinpocetine/piracetam or oxiracetam and Hydergine (P & H in small doses, don't worry)."

LR
Renton, Washington

"Have had slight increase in short-term memory capacity while taking Ginkgo and choline. I hope to experiment with more smart drugs/nutrients."

ME
San Antonio, Texas

"I have been taking piracetam and Hydergine for a period of two months. However, unfortunately, I have not noticed any improvement in my memory whatsoever. Neither have I noticed any improvement in my concentration. I really had expected excellent results from these two smart drugs after reading your book. I am sorry to have to give you the bad news that the smart drugs don't work on everybody.

"Perhaps you might be able to tell me what I am doing wrong. I am taking 2400 mg of piracetam in 800 mg doses three times a day, and 15 mg of Hydergine in five mg doses three times a day also."

FM
Ballwin, Missouri

Comment: Reread the sections of *Smart Drugs & Nutrients* and this book regarding the synergistic effects of smart drugs, and the "inverted-U-shaped dose-response curve." You are almost certainly taking enough piracetam and Hydergine to push you into the down side of the dose-response curve. Too much is too much, not enough is not enough, and just right is just right!

"A friend (went) to Mexico and was successful in getting three bottles of piracetam 800 mg. I have now tried them for two days. The first day I tried the 'attack dose' suggested by one of the writers in one of the publications, and I noticed intense concentration for a several hour period following that dosage of nine pills.

"Today, I have gone to the recommended dosage of divided doses of two pills three times daily, and I have again noticed a dramatic ability to concentrate deeply on the topics I'm working on. Hopefully, this is not just an effect similar to a placebo effect.

"I'll keep you informed. As an interesting sidelight, the Mexican pharmacist asked my friend for a prescription, and she had none. He told her he'd give her a single bottle of 30 pills for $15 if she'd give him an additional $50, and three bottles for $45 if she'd give him an additional $100. She knew that I was interested in trying the pills so she paid him what he asked. Therefore, $45 in pills cost $145.

"I've mailed an order to the pharmacy in San Ysidro, but I have heard nothing back yet."

Anonymous

Comment: Your friend should have walked out the door and gone to the next pharmacy. This is the first time we have heard of this kind of banditry. No prescription is required for piracetam in Mexico. Best of luck with the San Ysidro pharmacy. Let us know if they are reliable. Our newsletter, *Smart Drug News*, regularly reviews reliable mail-order sources.

"I just started taking Pearson and Shaw's IQ Plus, CoQ$_{10}$ and choline on a daily basis. I notice that I am much more alert, need less sleep, and have more energy."

RSK
Charleston, West Virginia

"After having a discussion with an FDA compliance officer, I know that I will want to make use of the directory of physicians that you offer. I never brought up the subject of nootropics, but instead posed as a patient worried about receiving necessary medications in the future. He brought them and your book up as 'problems' and reasons to tighten the policy. Anyway, I'm sure you've heard it all before. To him (and the FDA), everything is always A-okay if controlled by doctors, though.

"P.S. I'm 23, with a bachelor's degree in chemistry."

RJ
Rolling Meadows, IL

Comment: The FDA's confiscatory policies forced this young man to lie to a government official in order to protect his own health. At the time of the fall of the U.S.S.R., the laws were so restrictive as to make every Soviet citizen a criminal just in order to survive. When the state wanted to eliminate a particular person, he or she could be conveniently arrested.

"I worked for about five years at a very small, highly competitive retail store. The hours were long (15-18/day), and stress levels were very high. Add to that a poor diet (junk food junkie) and a boss who was so afraid of being wrong, she'd mess with people's heads if necessary. Needless to say, I was a wreck after all of this. I lived in a haze, never feeling fully alert. I could no longer discern

whether what I remembered was true or false. My short term memory was near non-existent. I felt like a zombie!

"Fortunately, a friend lent me his copy of Mondo 2000, *which had an excerpt from* SD&N. *I immediately decided to give some of these substances a try — anything to feel real again. The only items you listed that I could get immediately were choline and B5.*

"It was amazing. Within a week, I felt on top of things again. My memory was much improved and I no longer felt like I'd just had a frontal lobotomy. After a few weeks, I reached a stable state, about where I was previous to this job. A few weeks of choline and B5 undid five years of damage! The only lasting affect from then is that I still have trouble focusing my concentration.

"I continue with the choline and B5 a year and a half later, and now supplement my diet with a multi-vitamin packet, which has a large amount of all the B vitamins. I need to stay sharp now as I am currently a full-time computer programmer and I'm going to school nights to finish my computer science degree. I am doing very well, in both programming and on my grades, and I know I owe it to you. Thanks!"

AT

"For years (I am now 44 years old) I have been ill and have spent a fortune on doctors. They have been very little help, and in fact have done more harm than good in a lot of respects.

"Your book, SD&N *has been a godsend.*

"In high school, I made poor grades because I couldn't concentrate or remember. My mental quickness and memory was horrible, and has been for years. My problems were compounded by fatigue.

"So far I have tried piracetam (800 mg two times/day) with Hydergine (1.5 mg two times/day) also centrophenoxine (250 mg one time/day) with 50 mg of Dilantin.

"I only tried this because I was desperate. But to my surprise, what a help it was! The Dilantin and centrophenoxine had a wonderful effect on me. I had more energy, was in a better mood

and I didn't have obsessive thoughts and compulsions as much as I used to. I can think and my mind is quicker and my memory improved greatly. Obviously, I had an increase in confidence.

"I have a difficult time getting Dilantin, although I do have an order placed overseas that hasn't arrived yet. A friend originally gave me a 10-day supply to try.

"I want to see a doctor who is aware of smart drugs. They help so much, and I really had no life without them. Believe me, I've tried everything and every kind of doctor you can think of. I need to try a few things to see which works best. But right now, I would put Dilantin and centrophenoxine on top of the list."

ML
Rockport, Texas

"I've tried to take note of some of the effects of the smart drugs I've used. I've tried to keep my views as objective as possible.

"Piracetam: Of all the drugs I tested, this caused me the greatest ill feeling. I had feelings of fatigue, tiredness and lethargy. I enclose a printout I received from InHome Health Services which lists some of these effects. In all doses that I tried, and with or without Hydergine, I found the effects negative. There was perhaps a tendency to make more obscure connections between ideas and discern trends more easily.

"Hydergine: Increased energy, concentration and alertness. Difficult to say if any improvement in memory. Side effects were a caffeine-like burn-out occasionally.

"Dilantin: Increased ability to focus on work and shut out distracting influences. No noticeable bad effects.

"Oxicebral (vincamine): Enhanced concentration, subtle stimulant effects. Increased susceptibility to motion sickness?

"Lucidril (centrophenoxine): stimulant effect very similar to caffeine. Less attention to detail? Good levels of motivation. Increased susceptibility to motion sickness.

"Deprenyl (selegiline): Increased concentration, energy and stamina, as a result an ability to cope with what would usually be

difficult situations. Enhanced confidence as a result. More focused, lessened anxiety? Fair motivation.

"Fipexide: For me, I found this drug phenomenal! I noticed increased concentration, awareness. Marked ability to shut out distracting influences (positive synergistic effect with Dilantin here). Lessened feelings of burnout, tiredness, and overloading academically. Enhanced motivation, especially for work at expense of other factors. Side effects: some reduction in emotions, happiness, sadness, anxiety. Maybe this is the price to pay for enhanced logical abilities?

"Vasopressin: Rapid increase in interest and motivation. Strangely enough, it didn't seem to have much effect when using Fipexide, as if I was already aroused as much as one can be."

JRAM
Sutton-in-Ashfield, England

"I've been using DMAE in combination with pantothenic acid and a good vegetarian multivitamin supplement for two months now. One of the first things I noticed was that I fall asleep faster and wake up with a clearer mind; I experience a much sounder, more restful sleep. I constantly feel more attuned to my creative potential. I've always been full of ideas, and now these ideas seem to manifest more readily.

"Another thing I've noticed is that I'm always in a great mood. I take things in stride and don't freak out constantly like I used to. For once, I truly feel alive and awake."

PW

"Pregnenolone has made our 14-year-old dog and two cats very youthful and smarter. It has changed my 78-year-old mother from a dizzy dame to a bright, cheerful, outgoing person."

DM
Hauula, Hawaii

"Several years ago, I followed Dr. Barnes' method of checking the thyroid (as described in Smart Drugs & Nutrients*). I checked mine for three weeks and my average temperature was 97 degrees.*

"When I reported this to my doctor, he dismissed this form of checking, and went only by the blood test, which showed me to be on the very low levels. For several years now, I have suffered with underlying depression almost daily, enough so that most of the time I never really felt up to accomplishing my duties nor doing any crafts, sewing etc. During this time I was experiencing family problems, so I thought this was probably why I was having so much depression on a continual basis. At that time also, I had my blood sugar checked and I showed to be border-line hypoglycemic. This I discovered before my test was taken.

"About one month ago, I decided to try an experiment. My mother is on a low dosage of thyroid of .075 mg, so I decided to try it and see if I would feel better. I have been on this dose for a month. Now I do not have any depression and my energy level has definitely increased to the point that I can accomplish many more things. I have been so thankful to the Lord that this seems to have been my problem all these years.

"I have a call into my physician today and if he doesn't allow me to continue, I have decided to find another doctor who will listen to me. I have acquired your directory of physicians for my area."

DM
Odessa, Texas

Comment: We applaud your initiative, and bemoan the state of a medical profession so hidebound and inflexible that you were forced to solve your problems without proper medical assistance. Call the American College of Advancement in Medicine (ACAM) (714-583-7666) for the name of a physician in your area who is likely to be familiar with Dr. Barnes' protocol.

"I've been taking Hydergine and piracetam (with choline) both separately and together for several months now. I generally take about 2400 mg piracetam and about three mg Hydergine per day,

after working up from lower dosages. Piracetam has a more pleasant effect, but Hydergine provides more energy. I've noticed an ability to stay in focus for longer periods of time with piracetam, and a sense of physical well-being. Both drugs tend to leave me drained and tired after about a week of continuous use. Sometimes I can't sleep more than six hours. Perhaps I should lower the dose, or take rest periods of no use.

"I've noticed that piracetam has the same effect on dreams that it does on waking attention. I have incredibly long, sometimes boring, dreams, and I can resume the same dream after waking up. They go on and on. Hydergine, on the other hand, makes my dreams more colorful and strange, sometimes gruesome, but I don't seem to mind at the time.

"Piracetam improved my typing speed (but not my spelling!)"

Anonymous

"For the past two months I have been taking piracetam (1200 mg) and Hydergine (Sandoz) daily. Any improvement in my mental capacity has certainly been subtle, but I do seem to have a greater ability to grasp complex and abstract concepts and ideas and to better retain verbal and written communications.

"Over a period of approximately 45 days, I took 300 mg [7 mg per day] of deprenyl. Unfortunately, I exhausted my supply of the drug just as I was beginning to notice a positive effect on my memory and on my ability to verbalize. It also seemed to have a very positive effect on my libido."

**JEB
Broomfield, Colorado**

"After using choline, I found I could go to parties and hear and concentrate on many different conversations in addition to mine. My eyesight also became very clear. Also, my vocabulary and

thinking became very concise...for example using the words 'like' and 'umm' [less often]."

EGE
Manhattan, Kansas

"I have used vasopressin and found it to be amazing."

BF
Glen Ellyn, Illinois

"I've been trying out some Hydergine and have experienced noticeable results. I found one result to be improved vision at night, which was unexpected. Mostly, I experience increased alertness and ability to keep track of details."

TL
Gainesville, Florida

"Ginkgo biloba and/or DMAE have helped me verbalize my thoughts into complete sentences. For years, I have had difficulty formulating words. I have better control of speaking."

AA
Plymouth, Minnesota

Computer Programming and Choline

"I've been taking choline w/ inositol and /or lecithin since the 70s. I'm a computer programmer, and this significantly improves my short term visual memory (I can 'hold more code in my head'). I could not perform at the same level otherwise.

"For me, the optimum dose is 300 100 mg choline with an equal amount of inositol about every three hours while I'm at work. Too much makes me spacey. I always use caffeine with it (or get lost in daydreams).

"Several years ago I tried 100 mg DMAE. It made me extremely jittery and destroyed my concentration. No positive effects noticed. I tried again, recently, with only 30 mg of a different brand: same results. I'm afraid these jitters (like way-too-much

caffeine) may coincide with an increase in blood pressure which I have to be careful of, so I'm not going to experiment with DMAE any more.

"Phosphatidylserine: Last week I started taking Life Extension International's Cognitex with 200 mg phosphatidylserine. The first time I took it, it actually improved my eyesight. I put on a pair of glasses with an older (weaker) prescription to be comfortable. I assume this improvement in vision is due to better alertness to the surroundings and resultant better focusing of the eyes. I like this stuff. I'm taking it at work. It seems to be a mild stimulant."

RR
Takoma Park, Maryland

"I tried DMAE, glutamic acid, choline/inositol, ginseng, and ginkgo. The results have been spectacular. Almost immediately, I had greater cognition, terrific memory recall, and an abundance of mental energy.

"I have already sent to several European drug companies listed in your book for their lists. I am anxious to experiment further, as I am now writing a novel and working on some short stories, and find the cognition-enhancement aspects of these substances to be extremely helpful.

"If possible, I would like your advice or opinion on this matter. I would also be grateful if you could refer me to other research in the field, if there is any.

"Thank you."

JDM
Gibbsboro, New Jersey

"I started taking piracetam in September of 1991. I began with an attack dose of 8000 mg. I then went on a high dose regimen for seven days of 2400 mg three times a day. I then quit for seven days and then began again with a standard dose of 800 mg three times daily. My current regimen is two weeks of 800 mg three times daily then two weeks off. This seems to be optimum.

"This regimen has produced the following effects: No physical phenomena whatsoever. I have been asked repeatedly, 'What does it do? What are the effects?' The only way I can describe it is that it is not physical in any way. There are no 'feelings' as when other agents are taken. The effect is purely subjective and cerebral. I describe it is as allowing access to vast banks of memory which were previously untappable.

"With this new memory, I have access to memories that were long-buried (I have confirmed, by conversation with my parents, childhood memories that I have only recently remembered). I seem to have more 'internal time', ie., I can resolve problems mentally in much less time than before.

"My retention is very complete now, and memorization by repetition requires only one to two repetitions before long-term memorization occurs. This is opposed to previous experience which required six or seven repetitions which would only insert the data into short-term memory. There also appears to be no 'muddling' of information. Visualization seems to have improved vastly, and dreams are now more vivid, although I think this is probably due to more positive events in my personal life. I have also noticed a large decrease in reaction time.

"Overall, I have noticed nothing but positive effects from piracetam. I have used vasopressin in conjunction with it on several intensive study situations, but do not have enough data to be able to report objectively on the results.

"For the record, I am a 29-year-old white male, 5'10" and 185 pounds. I am in good health. I have recently (since the regimen began) dropped from being a heavy smoker (more than 1.5 packs daily) to a light smoker (less than one half pack daily) with intention to quit within three months. I have changed from a high-cholesterol, high-fat, red-meat-every-day diet, to a low-fat, low-cholesterol, red-meat-once-a-week diet. I have also begun a graduated exercise program. These changes have had the subjective effect of obviating the effects of piracetam, but are probably due to the reduced body stress."

MS
Irving, Texas

"I've experimented extensively with phenytoin (Dilantin). I use it any time I have to be in top form after not getting enough sleep, or if I need more stamina, or if events leave me emotionally upset without the opportunity to make things better.

"Several years ago I was in Thailand, trekking in the mountains north of Chang Mai. I live at sea level, and suddenly I was walking though the opium fields a mile up! I was starting to feel exhausted, and we still had a good climb ahead of us. I popped a 50 mg Infatab chewable dilantin in my mouth, let it melt, and within two minutes noticed how much better I felt. I began to walk faster than everyone in our party.

"We reached our destination, a tiny village of the Aka people. I felt great, and thoroughly enjoyed our visit. Some of my trekmates were too exhausted to enjoy the Aka's hospitality and humor.

"Late at night, the Aka chief offered opium to those of us still awake. Our guides and one of our party smoked three or four bowls each and quickly fell asleep. I smoked some, and, oddly, felt nothing. After 17 bowls and some wide-eyed stares from the chief, I decided I had better quit even though all I felt was a slight itch in my skin. I have wondered ever since if the dilantin blocked the effects of the opium.

"I went to sleep two hours later, feeling a deep sense of well-being. I woke up feeling refreshed and ready-to-go the next morning. My trek-mates refused my offer of Dilantin and felt exhausted all day (they were medical people, and knew better than to try a non-recreational drug without a prescription!)"

LM-W
Amsterdam, Netherlands

Comment: You're right. The Dilantin may have interfered with the effects of the opium. We have had anecdotal reports of Dilantin blocking the effects of marijuana and completely blocking the effects of LSD only six hours after the LSD was administered. Stick to smart drugs, they're safer.

"I have been a life-extension and smart-drug proponent for several years. I have been using choline chloride and DMAE for about five years now, and am certain that much of my improved memory functions over the past few years are a result of this regimen. I also use L-phenylalanine, caffeine and occasionally some ephedra."

MAJ
Bowling Green, Ohio

"I am a 52-year-old man. My physician has me on 50 mg of DHEA per day. One month ago, I started 250 mg of DMAE and five mg of Vinpocetine. The results have been incredible. My memory, concentration, alertness, lack of depression, and increased energy have shown remarkable improvement. (Unfortunately, it hasn't helped my typing or spelling.)

"My father started taking the same doses of DHEA and Vinpocetine on Christmas day. Believe me, the difference in his mood, lack of depression, and memory have been quite noticeable."

Anonymous

"After taking piracetam for six months (1.2 grams/day, generic), I added 4.5 mg Hydergine (Sandoz) to my daily regimen, and it enlightened me to the inverted-U dose-response curve. I engage in a weekly variety of mental tests (stabilized after three years), which in addition to real-world indicators allow me to optimize dosages quite effectively. Within one week of Hydergine introduction, my test scores began falling slightly, resettling six weeks later at lower levels than before therapy in all tests. Further, I felt continually fatigued and unmotivated.

"Armed with research on inverse-response and synergistic combinations, I readjusted my doses, finally settling on 2.25 mg Hydergine and 400-800 mg piracetam, the latter varying with levels of physical activity (weight-lifting days require higher dose, discovered separately.) Subsequently, my testing performance

eclipsed all previous levels by measurable and consistent (three consecutive months) margins.

"Best of luck publishing Smart Drugs II, *as I'm sure it will create quite a stir!"*

JGVV
Temperance, MI

The Smart Drugs Conference of 1991

An international scientific conference, held in October, 1991 in Monte Carlo, brought together many of the world's top researchers in the use of smart drugs for treatment of mental decline. Of course, it was not called a "smart drugs" conference — some scientists seem to avoid the phrase "smart drugs" the way a high-school biology teacher avoids the word "sex." The conference was called "Treatment of Age-Related Cognitive Dysfunction: Pharmacological and Clinical Evaluation." Presenters came to the conference from Belgium, France, Sweden, Italy, Germany, Portugal, the United Kingdom, and the United States.

The conference covered causes of cognitive impairment, methods of diagnosis, methods of testing the many drugs being used to improve cognition, and discussion of regulatory problems for smart-drug research. Here are some of the highlights from the 15 presentations:

A New Disease: Normal Aging

Dr. Kathleen C. Raffaele of the National Institute on Aging (one of the National Institutes of Health) and colleagues presented a paper on the concept of age-associated memory impairment (AAMI). In *Smart Drugs & Nutrients* we referred to the broader condition "age-related mental decline" (ARMD) (see the graph below). Dr. Raffaele made a strong case that normal cognitive loss with age should be considered a disease. There are well-documented age-associated decrements in many aspects of cognitive performance including perceptual speed, choice reaction time, visuospatial abilities, word fluency, some types of memory, and some types of attention. Raffaele emphasized the importance of treating not only clinical conditions but also normal age-associated memory impairment.

We realize that it may be disconcerting to consider that we all suffer from a disease called AAMI. However, we might be better off if the FDA thought this way. Currently, the FDA's charter allows approval of drugs only for the treatment of formally defined diseases. Therefore, no drugs get approved for simply improving the quality of life (or enhancing the performance or improving the sex lives) of otherwise healthy people. FDA approval for a drug for recreation or relaxation is currently out of the question.

If AAMI is classified as a disease, the pharmaceutical-regulatory system will develop and approve drugs for this condition. The financial incentives could impel a revolution in medicine.

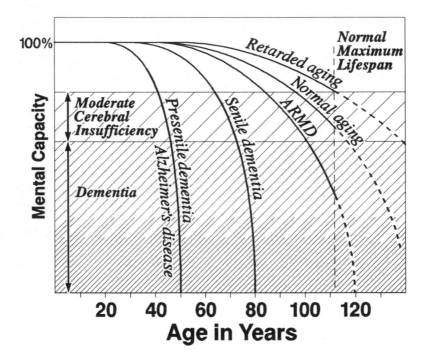

FDA Physician Speaks Out Against FDA Roadblocks to Aging Treatment

Dr. Paul Leber, of FDA's Office of New Drug Evaluation, candidly discussed the regulatory red tape which keeps the lid on smart-drug development in the U.S. Leber was careful to state that the opinions expressed in his presentation were his own, and did not represent the FDA's official position. We congratulate Dr. Leber on his courage to speak out when his job is on the line.

Leber pointed out that FDA has not taken a formal position on drugs for the treatment of age-related cognitive dysfunction. He understated that, "There is little encouragement given to the development of products intended to enhance the normal human condition." He cited the large number of drugs approved to treat depression and noted — perhaps with some irony — that the FDA has *never* approved any psychoactive euphoriant substance designed to "lift the spirits of a euthymic [non-depressed] individual after a tough day at the office." In fact, under current law, such drugs are considered to be drugs of abuse.

Leber continued, "The contrasting effects of this unofficial public standard are illustrated by the fact that human recombinant growth hormone is approved for the treatment of certain forms of dwarfism, a developmental disease, but not for the treatment of children whose heights place them in the lower tail of the population distribution."

Leber believes that "drug products intended to improve the performance of the healthy...will face barriers to their approval not experienced by products advanced for the treatment of what society accepts as a bona fide illness." He suggested, however, that acceptance of the concept of AAMI may, to some degree, lower these barriers.

Diagnosing Age-Related Memory Impairment

Dr. Thomas Crook of Memory Assessment Clinics, Inc., suggested that one of the problems with the acceptance of AAMI as a disease category is the lack of a standardized diagnostic method. He then reviewed specific methods to assess the clinical efficacy of smart drugs in subjects with AAMI. Signs of AAMI include difficulty recalling extensive verbal or numerical information, and difficulty learning and recalling new information quickly or in the face of distraction. He presented data from his recent studies on phosphatidylserine and ondansetron which showed clear improvement in subjects with AAMI (see the chapters on these drugs). Dr. Crook believes that tests sensitive enough to detect and measure the slow mental decline in normal aging do now exist. The presentation

Proportion of Subjects with Verbal Memory Impairment

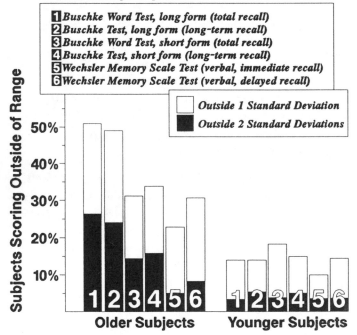

1 Buschke Word Test, long form (total recall)
2 Buschke Test, long form (long-term recall)
3 Buschke Word Test, short form (total recall)
4 Buschke Test, short form (long-term recall)
5 Wechsler Memory Scale Test (verbal, immediate recall)
6 Wechsler Memory Scale Test (verbal, delayed recall)

Outside 1 Standard Deviation
Outside 2 Standard Deviations

ended with an optimistic statement that age-related cognitive deficits can be improved by pharmacologic treatment.

Multiple Treatments for Memory

Professor Kjell Fuxe of the Karolinska Institute in Stockholm, and colleagues, discussed the alterations of neural communication that take place with aging, different types of synaptic transmission, and how more specific drugs could be developed to reverse these changes. They recommended that patients with learning and memory disorders receive memory training in addition to receiving drug treatment for cognition enhancement. Finally, they emphasized that increased formation of free radicals in the central nervous system (CNS) may lead to gene damage and a disregulation of gene function. This can result in an abnormal increase or decrease of gene transcription

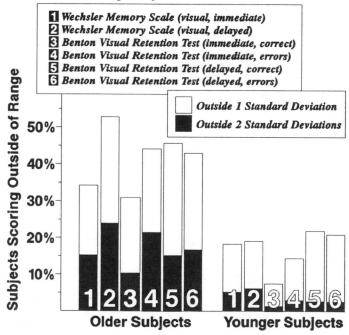

Proportion of Subjects with Visual Memory Impairment

1 *Wechsler Memory Scale (visual, immediate)*
2 *Wechsler Memory Scale (visual, delayed)*
3 *Benton Visual Retention Test (immediate, correct)*
4 *Benton Visual Retention Test (immediate, errors)*
5 *Benton Visual Retention Test (delayed, correct)*
6 *Benton Visual Retention Test (delayed, errors)*

☐ *Outside 1 Standard Deviation*
■ *Outside 2 Standard Deviations*

Subjects Scoring Outside of Range

Older Subjects   Younger Subjects

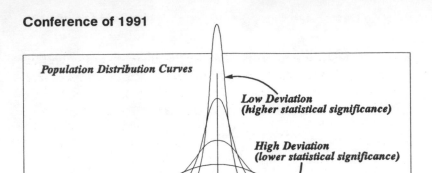

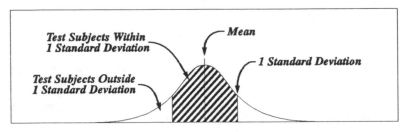

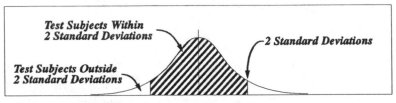

Definition: Standard Deviation and Statistical Significance
In the top illustration, bell-shaped distributions of data values vary from high
deviation (broad, flat curve) to low-deviation (high, narrow curve). Within a
distribution (middle illustration), statisticians mathematically determine a
standard deviation which is used to separate "hump" and "fringe" data points.

for various biologically-active molecules, such as
neuropeptides, neurotrophic factors, and their receptors. They
discussed methods of reducing levels of free radicals and
increasing levels of free-radical scavengers within the CNS
including increasing cerebral blood flow, improving glucose
metabolism, and enhancing mitochondrial function.

Theories of How Smart Drugs Work

Dr. Walter E.Müller, of the Central Institute of Mental Health
in Mannheim, Germany, maintained that cognition enhancers

were generally much more effective in older than in younger people. This holds true for compounds of different classes like piracetam (the standard nootropic drug), pyritinol (a "metabolic enhancer"), and phosphatidylserine (a synaptic enhancer). He suggested that these drugs work by correcting for age-related changes in the brain, specifically by restoring the loss of cholinergic and NMDA receptor systems to more youthful levels.

Müller reported significant cognition improvement with each of the three above-mentioned smart drugs. Furthermore, he found that all three resulted in increased cholinergic receptor activity even though the drugs are in different pharmacological subclasses. Müller cited studies by others which documented positive effects of *Ginkgo biloba* extract and Hydergine.

Piracetam Reverses Alcohol-Induced Brain Degeneration

Portugal's Dr. Fernando Brandão and his colleagues noted that long-term alcohol consumption induces structural CNS changes identical to those caused by aging. They looked at the ability of piracetam to reverse the degenerative activity of alcohol in rat brains. The researchers presented their findings that piracetam had a neuroprotective effect, stabilized neuronal membranes, increased neuronal protein synthesis, showed anti-oxidant properties, improved neuronal catabolic capability, and dramatically reduced lipofuscin formation.

The Seven Classes of Smart Drugs

An excellent survey of the various classes of cognition-enhancing agents currently under evaluation was presented by Dr. C. G. Gottfries, of the University of Göteborg in Sweden. These classes are: 1) vasodilators; 2) nootropics; 3) neuro-transmitter modulators/replacements; 4) nerve growth factors; 5) essential nutrients; 6) aluminum chelators; and 7) miscellaneous substances (which included phosphatidylserine, acetyl-L-carnitine, and gangliosides). Studies of drugs in each of these classes were briefly discussed.

Piracetam Plus Cognitive Training

Dr. Walter Deberdt, of UCB Pharmaceuticals, reported on several placebo-controlled studies in which subjects with AAMI were given various doses of piracetam in combination with cognitive training. He found the combined treatments to be synergistic.

Animal Models for Aging in Humans

France's Dr. Roger Porsolt and his colleagues reviewed some current approaches to evaluation of cognition enhancers in animals. They pointed out that since no animal model is currently accepted for Alzheimer's disease, the best available animal model for the aging human is the aging animal. Their aim was to search for behavioral phenomena in animals which show clear analogies with aging humans. They then discussed the complex problem of selecting an appropriate means to evaluate cognitive performance in animals, and reviewed the advantages and disadvantages of various standard screening tests. Studies were cited for each test in which cognition-enhancing drugs had been evaluated.

Conclusion

While the FDA publicly maintains that smart drugs don't exist (or are dangerous), scientists are developing second-generation smart drugs and improved methods of measuring the subtle cognitive deficits of age-related mental decline. Better measurement systems will make evaluation of new smart drugs easier.

References

Mendlewicz J and Racagni G [Eds.]. *Treatment of Age-Related Cognitive Dysfunction: Pharmacological and Clinical Evaluation.* Karger, Basel, 1992. ISBN: 3-8055-5551-2, 154 pages, $111.25.

Part III:

Questions & Answers

Part III: Questions & Answers

Questions & Answers

After the release of *Smart Drugs & Nutrients*, our readers began writing and calling with every imaginable question. We were swamped and, unfortunately, many people's questions went unanswered.

Steven Fowkes, and the staff of the Cognitive Enhancement Research Institute (CERI), responded by publishing a question-and-answer section in the Institute's newsletter, *Smart Drug News*. The Q&A section has consistently been the most popular section of *Smart Drug News*. What follows are selected excerpts from this section. Some questions have been grouped together. We've also added a few updates where necessary. The initials at the end of some of the questions indicates the specific author answering the question. WD is Ward Dean, JM is John Morgenthaler, SWF is Steven Fowkes, and TMH is T. Mike Hardy, Assistant Editor of *Smart Drug News*. Initials of the questioners have been omitted.

Smart Drug News is published 10 times annually by CERI. You can subscribe by mailing in the tear-out subscription card at the front of this book with your check or credit card information. The subscription price is $44 per year ($46 Canada/Mexico, $55 overseas). Or subscribe by calling CERI at 415-321-CERI (415-321-2374).

The material in this section, like the rest of the book, is indexed. If you are interested in information on a certain substance or condition you can look it up in the index and there may be some pointers into this section.

Question: *Someone on the* Phil Donahue Show *said that there are no studies where smart drugs were given to normal, healthy humans. Is this true?*

Answer: No. There have been many studies of various smart drugs that have used normal, healthy, non-demented people.

Frankly, we've been surprised by the number of scientists in the field who are also unfamiliar with the wealth of research with normal people. Because of the importance of this kind of research, this book and a regular department in *Smart Drug News* feature normal, healthy human studies of smart drugs. See the "Normal, healthy humans" listing in the Index for a list of these studies.

Question: *Are smart drugs legal?*

Answer: Many smart drugs are commonly prescribed in the U.S. for other uses. FDA law prohibits drug manufacturers from publicizing research showing that a drug has uses other than the "FDA-approved" ones. The FDA only approves drugs for treating disease. "Normal" age-associated memory impairment (AAMI) is not considered a disease by the FDA. The FDA is not interested in approving a drug developed solely for the purpose of improving mental function in normal people — a use the FDA considers to be recreational.

Some researchers and physicians are now asking the medical community and the FDA to recognize AAMI as a disease — a disease we all get as we age. Scientists have established that smart drugs are effective in treating AAMI. It is time for the U.S. government to recognize AAMI and approve smart drugs for the preser- vation of our most precious national resources — the wisdom, productivity, experience and spirits of our older people.

Question: *One of my friends said that smart drugs are perfectly safe. One of the doctors on TV said they are dangerous. Who's right?*

Answer: Neither. Nothing is perfectly safe. Smart drugs, as a class, have among the fewest side effects of any pharmaceu-ticals. Hydergine, for example, has only one contraindication listed in the *Physicians Desk Reference*: hypersensitivity to the drug. The only adverse effect listed is mild gastric distress, which is rare to non-existent. It has been prescribed millions of times over the last thirty years without any serious problems.

Piracetam has no known side effects or contraindications and has been prescribed millions of times in Europe and Asia.

Question: *Are smart drugs safe? What kind of medical supervision is required? What tests do you recommend?*

Answer: The safety, medical supervision and tests that we recommend depend upon which smart drug or drugs are being taken. Some drugs, like piracetam, acetyl-L-carnitine (ALC), phosphatidylserine (PS), and Hydergine, are so safe that we believe they should be afforded over-the-counter status in the U.S. The same can be said for most of the nutrients which influence brain function, like phenylalanine, tryptophan, pyroglutamate, choline or DMAE (dimethylaminoethanol). This is not to say that they cannot be abused or cannot cause serious problems when used inappropriately. Despite the safety of most of these substances, taking an entire bottle of smart drugs or 10-1000 times a normal dose of smart nutrients could be toxic, especially for children. (Too much salt, aspirin, Tylenol, or even water can also be toxic). *Caution and consideration are essential.*

Thus, medical supervision is always recommended for smart-drug use. Since most drugs are metabolized by the liver, and are excreted by the kidneys, tests of the functioning of these organs are recommended. Before embarking on a smart drug regimen, ask your physician to perform the following blood tests: uric acid, blood urea nitrogen (BUN), and serum creatinine (for testing kidney function); and SGOT, SGPT and GGTP (to evaluate the liver).

These standard blood tests can pinpoint short-term toxic reactions before they might be noticed subjectively. These tests should be repeated at periodic intervals — the frequency determined by your physician based on your personal body chemistry and the drug/nutrient combinations you may be taking. Although smart drugs as a class are among the safest substances known (with few or no known adverse effects or toxicities), combinations have not been well tested and medical monitoring is prudent and strongly recommended.

Question: *I saw James McGaugh on TV saying smart drugs don't work. He was also an incredible grouch. What's his story?*

Answer: Dr. McGaugh is director of the Center for the Neurobiology of Learning and Memory at the University of California, Irvine. McGaugh has for many years explored the mysteries of thought, memory and cognition in his laboratory. Our search of the medical database turned up an astounding 141 papers attributed to Dr. McGaugh on the subjects of memory, learning, IQ, cognition, senility, Alzheimer's disease or dementia! The earliest paper attributed to McGaugh is from 1966, but the database only carries papers dating back to 1966.

Before the smart drug media circus hit the fan, Dr. McGaugh spoke candidly on BBC's *Horizon*, "In the laboratory there already exists a large number of drugs that can improve memory in laboratory animals. That's a very easy experiment to do." (Interested viewers may want to call the producers of Horizon's sister show, *Nova*, WGBH/Boston, at 617-492-2777, to request that they air the *Horizon* show called "Food For Thought".)

McGaugh continued, "In my laboratory as well as many other laboratories throughout the world, we've shown that memory in rats and mice can be improved by a number of drugs that are currently available." Sitting in the glow of a computer screen, Dr. McGaugh opined, "Human memory is like animal memory, in terms of the basic mechanism, the physiological machinery. Now, the content is likely to be quite different; that is, the things you think about and I remember are different from the things my rat remembers. But the mechanisms that enable the memory in both cases, I'm going to assert, are the same."

Soon after Horizon aired every media person with a pencil and a telephone credit card started calling McGaugh seeking the scoop on smart drugs. The good doctor began to wax combative. He told a journalist from Health magazine, "*No*-otropics. That's the perfect name for these, they have *no* effect!"

There are at least 10 million regular piracetam users in the world. That's a lot of "no-otropic" effect.

Washington Post reporter Karen Marrero must have been nonplused when Dr. McGaugh told her he was "nauseated" by the promotion of the substances in *Smart Drugs & Nutrients*. He hurled, "There is nothing in that book that should be taken. N-O-T-H-I-N-G, nothing. And every scientist I know in the field shares this view."

Perhaps Dr. McGaugh does not know researchers Turan Itil ("There is no doubt that these drugs increase cognitive performance; among others, attention and concentration. Due to the results of better information gathering, they may have increased IQ."), Keith Wesnes ("We've shown in a number of populations from young people to healthy older to demented patients that drugs can improve various aspects of mental efficiency."), Raymond Bartus ("They're relatively safe and they may improve quality of life"), Stephen Schoenthaler (see our chapter on vitamins), or Dr. József Knoll ("Alzheimer's disease patients need to be treated daily with 10 mg deprenyl from diagnosis until death").

Before the Washington Post's hapless writer could get off the phone, the crusty-but-lovable Dr. McGaugh attempted the final word on smart drugs, "They are all experimental drugs." If that's true, the whole world outside of the U.S. is one hell of a big laboratory. Piracetam is sold in 85 countries, and piracetam and Hydergine are sold over the counter in Belgium, Mexico, Thailand, Italy, and many others. These drugs account for billions of dollars in sales annually worldwide.

So why is Dr. McGaugh upset about *Smart Drugs & Nutrients*? He told Jerry Stahl, in an interview with *Playboy* magazine, "The book *Smart Drugs & Nutrients* is not a legitimate science book. It's not a balanced view of the literature in the field." We agree that *Smart Drugs & Nutrients* is not a "legitimate science book." It is a book about legitimate science. It is a popular treatment of the field that makes reference to over 250 scientific papers. It is also a how-to guide for people who wish to apply this science to themselves. Legitimate science books with names like *Treatment of Age-Related Cognitive Dysfunction: Pharmacological and Clinical Evaluation* are not useful for non-scientists.

We would also like to respond to the statement that our book is not a balanced view of the literature. The word "balanced" seems to imply that we are required to give all points of view, no matter how flawed, equal weight. Our objective was to review the literature and present what seemed to be the best argument. And we tried to "balance" the research done overseas with that done in the U.S.

Dr. McGaugh also told Playboy that our "whole approach is about as serious as astrology. That's why so many of my colleagues are bitter and angry. It cheapens our field."

We can certainly understand if, after a lifetime of dedication to the research, Dr. McGaugh is frustrated with upstarts like us basking in the limelight (compared to old-timer McGaugh nearly everyone in this field is an upstart.) If this is the case, we would like to take this opportunity to humbly apologize to James L. McGaugh.

We would also like to state that we are serious. We are here for the long haul. And we plan to be surfing the edge of smart drugs technology when everyone in America (but, presumably, Dr. McGaugh) is using performance enhancers.

Dr. McGaugh is a pioneer in the smart drug field, a real mover and a shaker. He deserves the respect and admiration of every person with an interest in this subject, regardless of whether that respect and admiration is ever reciprocated.

Mendlewicz J and Racagni G [Eds.]. *Treatment of Age-Related Cognitive Dysfunction: Pharmacological and Clinical Evaluation.* Karger, Basel, 1992. ISBN: 3-8055-5551-2, 154 pages, $111.25!

Question: *When I first bought the* Smart Drugs & Nutrients *book in the fall, I sent a SASE to get the directory of physicians.*

Unfortunately, at that time, all of the doctors on the list were from the West Coast. Has the list grown to include doctors in my area (New England)?

Answer: Yes. The Northeast is now represented on our directory of physicians.

Question: *I received your directory of physicians in March and attempted to contact one of the physicians on the list. I got a very cold reception from his receptionist and was told that they have been trying to get his name off your list. I think it is wise to remove his name from your list until such time as he requests to be re-enrolled. It is my belief that CERI cannot afford to alienate the few members of the medical community who are liberal enough to consider proactive health. I hope that a letter will be sent to the physician apologizing for the misunderstanding and notifying him that his name will be removed from the list.*

Answer: We were very concerned about your report and spoke to the physician's staff immediately. We were unable to confirm a problem. We were told that the doctor does want to be listed, and has not tried to have his name removed from the list. The discrepancy between your experience and our inquiry makes us wonder if you may have called at a bad time, got a disgruntled employee, or something even more bizarre. You might want to try again.

Thanks for the report. We appreciate your thoughtfulness and consideration in letting us know right away. If you try again, let us know how it goes. **SWF**

Comment: *My physician is willing to write me prescriptions for cognition-enhancing pharmaceuticals, but he really isn't well-educated in the interactions between the various drugs.*

Response: Your physician is not alone. Although few studies have been conducted on interactions between various smart drugs and other prescriptions and over-the-counter medications, reports of adverse reactions have been extremely rare. This is probably due to the overwhelming safety of most smart drugs. The possibility always exists, however, that a previously untried combination, dosage, or a person with a unique bio-chemical reaction may result in a previously unreported adverse reaction. This is why we recommend physician monitoring, and that untried medications be initiated at low dosages, and increased gradually. **WD**

Question: *I'm having problems finding a physician who will write me a prescription for Hydergine and vasopressin. The docs I've seen react with alarm and say that there is no medical need for me to use these medications. I just get blank stares when I mention cognitive enhancement. Even physicians on the CERI directory of physicians react this way. Any suggestions?*

Answer: Unfortunately, you're not going to get a prescription for these drugs from the vast majority of physicians for a number of reasons. First, physicians are trained to treat disease. Most physicians consider the taking of medications by normal people to be a "recreational use" and will probably try to discourage you (as you have found out). Second, they are concerned about peer pressure and peer review (i.e., other physicians looking askance over their shoulders at such nonstandard therapy). Third, you cannot expect your physician to prescribe such drugs if you want to pay for the visit with medical insurance (medical insurance is to pay for treatments for *disease* — and so far, age-associated memory impairment is not considered a disease by most insurance companies). Fourth, physicians generally have a tendency to be "down on things they're not up on." Few physicians have much knowledge about cognition-enhancing drugs.

So — what do you do? First, as you mentioned, try physicians on the CERI directory of physicians. Let us know if you have a problem with a particular physician.

Do not expect to see him one time and get a "lifetime refillable prescription" for Hydergine or other smart drugs. Because of medical ethics and regulations which require physicians to monitor and evaluate their patients at reasonable intervals (and their need to pay the rent), most physicians will prescribe a three- to six-month supply. At that time, you will need to pay for another office visit for another prescription, and perhaps a blood test (to monitor liver and kidney function) at the least.

Make sure to tell both the physician and the receptionist that you will be paying cash, and will not be submitting the bill to an insurance company (unless you are being treated for an illness).

Another source of physicians is the American College of Advancement in Medicine (ACAM) (714-583-7666). ACAM physicians are among the most open-minded in the country, and pride themselves on staying abreast of new developments which enhance their patients' health. They will generally read health information provided by their patients, and are more likely to try a therapy that a patient requests than other physicians (if the therapy appears safe and likely to be of benefit).

If the ACAM physician in your area is not aware of smart drugs, provide him with a copy of *Smart Drugs & Nutrients* and ask him to call me if he has any questions (he has my number in his ACAM Directory).   **WD**

More: Most orthodox physicians are reluctant to prescribe drugs for what they believe are elective purposes. The dominant view in the medical profession is that drugs are for treatment of disease, and "normal" people don't need them. This view — that if you are not sick you are well — is based on a simplistic and unscientific understanding of health and disease. There are, in fact, just as many levels or degrees of health as there are of disease.

Even when patients are not well, doctors are loath to admit that you have a disease they do not know about or understand. Rather than say they don't know what's wrong with you, a large percentage of doctors will call your "disease" psychosomatic or mental in origin. Rather than seeking an understanding of your condition beyond their knowledge, they refer you to a psychiatrist.

Open-minded physicians willing to work with a patient outside the limitations of peer-regulated medicine are rare resources. Don't abuse them. Work with them within the limitations imposed by their reactionary peers, judgment-hungry lawyers, malpractice-averse insurance companies, and punitive medical boards.

When seeking a physician, remember that physicians are trained to conduct professional relationships with their patients. This means a long-term relationship based on professional responsibility for your medical care. It is generally a bad mistake to approach a physician for the primary purpose of getting a prescription. Physicians resent being treated like drug pushers.

While it is legal by federal law for doctors to write prescriptions for unapproved uses, it is against state licensing regulations for doctors to practice medicine which is not recognized as appropriate by their peers. In other words, medicine is regulated like a medieval guild. This poses ticklish problems for doctors who think for themselves.

Because peer-review medicine tends to be mediocre, state-of-the-art medicine is often unrecognized as such by other doctors. Doctors who work with smart drugs, life extension, holistic medicine, preventive medicine, or nutritional medicine are putting their medical practices, and their security, at risk. They are often willing to do that with their best patients, but can be extremely reluctant to do that with somebody they don't yet know, who walks off the street asking for drugs.

Eventually, cognitive technology will become incorporated into mainstream medicine and smart drugs will become as accepted as ibuprofen and aspirin are today. But at that time, some other medical technology will be state-of-the-art and unrecognized by mainstream medicine. That's the way "progress" progresses.

When establishing a relationship with a physician, interview him as to his philosophy about the practice of medicine. Find out whether he will work with you in the way you want. Is he willing to work with you in counteracting age-associated memory impairment? Is he willing to prescribe drugs for unapproved uses if they provide you with a benefit? Is he affordable? Physicians can charge better than $100/hour. Is he willing to listen to your point of view? What does his staff think of your goals? What do his patients think about the doctor's services?   **SWF**

Question: *Which of the smart drugs is best to start with?*

Answer: This is a question we're frequently asked. the answer is — it depends. Unfortunately, there is no smart drug that works well for everyone. Nor is there any known way to test in advance who will respond best to which smart drug. Therefore, the use of smart drugs remains empiri- cal, and the choice of which drug/substance to start with is a very individualized one. For example, many users of cognitive-enhancement substances prefer to use "natural" (non-drug) substances. For them, the best substances to start with are: 1) over-the-counter nutrients from health food stores, like dimethylaminoethanol (DMAE), Gingko biloba, or phenylalanine; or 2) pre-prepared combination products containing neurotransmitter precursors like choline, tyrosine, phenylalanine, pyroglutamate, etc. For those who have a cooperating, knowledgeable physician, Hydergine and vasopressin may be tried initially. For those who live close to the Mexican border, or who can order from overseas pharmacies, well-tested drugs that can be highly recommended for first-time use include piracetam and deprenyl.   **WD**

Question: *Where can I get smart drugs?*

Answer: Your physician can prescribe smart drugs, like Hydergine, that are available in the U.S. CERI maintains a directory of physicians working in this field. For a copy of this directory, send a self-addressed, stamped envelope and $2 to CERI, P.O. Box 4029, Menlo Park, CA 94026-4029. *Physicians: if you'd like to be listed, please send us a brief description of your practice.* (Please see the tearout card at the front of this book.)

Many smart drugs are available over-the-counter overseas and in Mexico. If you can get to the border yourself, you can walk across, take a taxi to the nearest pharmacy, and buy many of the drugs you want. The customs inspectors will allow you to bring back a "reasonable" quantity of most drugs (approximately a

3-month supply). Drugs that are controlled in the United States (*i.e.* narcotics, sedatives and anabolic steroids) will probably be confiscated. To practically guarantee that you will not be hassled, it may be a good idea to have your physician write prescriptions for the drugs you intend to purchase. Although the prescription is not necessary to buy the drugs in Mexico, it will virtually eliminate any potential problems you might otherwise have in bringing them back into the United states. (Also, see Appendix A on sources for smart drugs.)

Question: *My wife (87 years old) has Alzheimer's disease. It seems the doctors have just given up, so we try any help available. You mention "nootropic" IQ boosters to aid memory, and smart pills. How and where can we get them?*

Answer: The basics are explained in *Smart Drugs & Nutrients* (copies are available from us). The FDA's personal importation policy is explained in Is All This Legal. Further information is available on an ongoing basis in our newsletter. Refer to *Smart Drug News* issue number two for our recommendations for use of the FDA's personal importation policy for unapproved drugs.

But before you purchase or use smart drugs, you need to establish professional medical supervision for yourself and your wife. The doctor can 1) guide you in selecting drugs, 2) protect you from adverse effects from drugs or drug combinations, 3) document improvements from drug use, and 4) assist in obtaining the drug through personal importation (if it is unavailable by prescription in the United States).

Although smart drugs can help to a variable degree in Alzheimer's disease, the specific clinical response depends on the patient and the drug(s) being used. Some patients experience little or no benefit with some drugs, and others experience very noticeable benefit. Keep trying until you find something that works.

Comment: *I thought you'd like to see the enclosed business card from a Mexican pharmacy closest to the border where I live. Although your Spanish may be better than mine, I can tell you* *that "¡Bienvenidos Paisanos!" roughly translates as everyone is welcome, and that "Farmacia del Niño" is the children's drugstore and "Farmacia de Dios" is the drugstore of God. Not such a bad place to get your smart drugs, eh? (I'll hold off making any seeing-God-on-smart-drugs jokes — until I do so myself, at least).*

Response: Great. Thanks for the tip, and the chuckle. We also liked the bullets on the card:
- The best service in town
- Top exchange rate every day
- The best stock in medicines and supplies
- Open seven days a week 8:00 a.m.-10:00 p.m.
- Three blocks from border
- VISA and MasterCard accepted

Question: *An article concerning smart drugs in* The Oregonian *stated that, "Since January, the FDA has been intercepting packages from six foreign companies selling various smart drugs." It did not state the names of the six companies, but I assume one of them is InHome Health Services, with whom I placed my first order (sounds like my money is down the drain). Short of a sojourn to Switzerland or Baja California, what viable alternatives do we now have for obtaining piracetam, centrophenoxine and other drugs that can't be prescribed in the U.S.?*

Answer: CERI is always adding new companies to its list of companies not on the FDA import alert list. The products you are interested in are readily available from most of them. Try contacting them for specific price and ordering information.

Question: *Can you send me names and addresses of current smart-drug suppliers from overseas? The few which I have been using appear to have been shut down or gone out of business.*

Answer: Yes, see our Sources section. New sources are listed in *Smart Drug News* as each issue is published, keeping our current subscribers up to date. They are also included in our product sources list which is updated on an ongoing basis to bring new subscribers up to date.

We appreciate hearing about sources from our subscribers. Often, you are the first people to know when a company goes out of business, or starts up business. Although the FDA's import alert does pose serious problems to companies doing business over the long run, the FDA is not very fast in assimilating information or reacting to it. Current companies are much more flexible and adapt to FDA tactics faster than the FDA adapts to them.

Comment: *If I could write a book disclaiming your book [Smart Drugs & Nutrients], I would. I feel you are responsible for my loss of approximately $68 sent to one of the overseas suppliers you mentioned in your book. I have sent copies of your book to the Compliance Officer at the Department of Health and Human Services who detained my order.*

Response: We are sorry that you may have lost your money. But you may not have. Your letter did not provide details of your experiences with the overseas supplier or the FDA's detention of your shipment. How long have you waited for a response from the supplier? Did you respond to the detention? Did the FDA destroy your order or did they ship it back to the supplier?

The FDA is not perfect in responding to letters, or even in notifying citizens of detentions or follow-up actions. In one case we know of, a subscriber was notified of the detention *weeks* after the deadline for response to the notification. The FDA, like other huge bureaucracies, is notoriously inefficient and capricious. Their decision to seize your drugs was solely their decision, not the overseas supplier, is not the publisher's, not John Morgenthaler's, not Dr. Ward Dean's, and not CERI's. The FDA's Personal Importation Policy, as listed in *Smart Drugs & Nutrients*, is the official policy of the FDA. It is not misrepresented. Just because the FDA will not follow their own policies when it suits them not to is the responsibility of nobody but the FDA.

If you cannot get satisfaction from the FDA despite legitimate use of the Personal Importation Policy, we suggest that you contact your Congressional representative and ask him/her to get involved in your case.

If you were not informed by the overseas supplier that you were accepting complete responsibility for the shipment, they might reship the order to you after it has been returned by U.S. Customs. If you do press your claim, the FDA might destroy the shipment rather than return it. Please discuss the detention issue with the supplier and find out what they will or will not do, and then let us know if you still have a grievance. The FDA has a reputation for trying to intimidate citizens. However, if you assert your legal rights, it is not uncommon for the FDA to "roll over" and do the right thing. **SWF**

Question: *In* Life Extension, *Pearson and Shaw warn that generic Hydergine may not have the same effectiveness as Sandoz Hydergine in various non-FDA-approved uses (as a smart drug). They claim that the biochemically significant distinction between alpha and beta forms of ergocryptine mesylate make the generic product different from Sandoz' Hydergine. Ward Dean doesn't mention this in* Smart Drugs & Nutrients. *Has further research been done on generic Hydergine? I've been taking generic Hydergine without much effect. Should I switch to Sandoz brand?*

Answer: At the time *Life Extension* was written, there were a number of nonstandardized formulations of ergoloid mesylates (the generic name for Hydergine) which used various proportions of the three drugs which comprise Hydergine. Since that time, however, the formulation has become standardized, and now all generic forms of Hydergine contain the same ratio of active ingredients. The bioavailability of the drug may be slightly less in the generics. However, taking a bit more of the generic is still more economical, considering the cost differential. For those for whom price is no object, I recommend Hydergine Liquid Capsules (or liquid Hydergine). These products have even higher bioavailability than the sublingual or oral tablets. **WD**

Question: *Someone told me that Hydergine doesn't work. What's the story?*

Answer: Hydergine has repeatedly demonstrated effectiveness in the treatment of many different conditions, from age-associated memory impairment to the prevention of oxygen-deprivation damage to the brains of automobile accident victims. Hydergine was the first drug to show efficacy against Alzheimer's disease. Hydergine's efficacy in treating dementias is as well-established as almost any other drug used for psychiatric disorders. As of 10 years ago, more than 20 double-blind placebo-controlled trials had been conducted to test Hydergine with senile dementias. All noted statistically significant improvements in behavioral and psychological parameters. Numerous favorable studies have been published since then.

One recent study, however, reported no improvement in 39 Alzheimer's patients who were treated with 1 mg Hydergine three times per day for six months. These negative results may be due to the disease having progressed beyond Hydergine's ability to help, or perhaps because an inadequate dosage of Hydergine was used. In an earlier study of patients with multi-infarct dementias or mental disturbances following strokes, Dr. Yoshikawa and colleagues demonstrated that a 6 mg per day dose was far superior to the standard 3 mg per day dose. The literature suggests that Hydergine treatment be started as early as possible in Alzheimer's patients.

Question: *The enclosed article by Dr. Lamb questions the use of Hydergine for memory enhancement citing research by Dr. Troy L. Thompson and colleagues at Jefferson Medical College in Philadelphia. What are your feelings about this research and Dr. Lamb's point of view?*

Answer: The article you sent is about a recent study in the New England Journal of Medicine, in which doses of three mg/day for six months were found to be ineffective in improving symptoms of eighty patients with Alzheimer's disease. The authors concluded that "Hydergine was ineffective as a treatment for Alzheimer's disease."

What the authors *really* proved, however, was that three mg per day is an *inadequate* dose for Alzheimer's disease. The question remains whether higher doses will benefit patients with Alzheimer's disease. Several earlier studies indicate that *higher* doses may be required to improve Alzheimer's disease. For example, a team of physicians at Stanford University [Yesavage, *et al.*, 1979] administered 6 mg of Hydergine each day to 14 hospitalized patients (aged 62-84) with senile deterioration. All of them had been treated for at least 4 months with 3 mg Hydergine per day, without noticeable improvement. However, after 12 weeks of treatment at the *higher* dose, seven of eleven surviving patients (three of the patients died due to unrelated causes) had shown *improvement*. One patient, who had been hospitalized for two years, improved so dramatically he was discharged from the hospital.

In another study in Japan, Yoshikawa and colleagues conducted a large double-blind study of Hydergine in 550 patients. They found that "almost half of the patients in the 6 mg group (48.9 per cent) showed a moderate to marked improvement, compared with only 17.9 per cent in the 3 mg group." Furthermore, they noted that "the superiority of a higher Hydergine dose was particularly pronounced in patients with heavy-headedness, sleep disturbances of various kinds, problems of concentration, loss of vigor, memory disturbances, and giddiness." They concluded that "the favorable effects of Hydergine on psychiatric, subjective and neurologic symptoms in patients with cerebrovascular disease are considerably increased when a higher dose is used," that "a daily dose of 3 mg may therefore be insufficient," and that "clinically relevant improvement may be obtained in more cases if the dose is increased to 6 mg per day." No adverse effects of the 6 mg dose were reported in either study. It is possible that even higher doses may be required for those who are severely demented. It is very interesting that the authors of the *New England Journal of Medicine* article which Dr. Lamb cited conveniently overlooked both of these beneficial studies. **WD**

Thompson TL, Filley II, Mitchell WD, Culig KM, Lo Verde M, and Byyny R. Lack of efficacy of Hydergine in patient's with Alzheimer's disease. *New England Journal of Medicine* 323: 445-448, 1990.

Yesavage JA, Hollister LE, and Burian E. Dihydroergotoxine [Hydergine]: 6 mg versus 3 mg dosage in the treatment of senile dementia. Preliminary report. *Journal of the American Geriatrics Society* 27: 80-2, 1979.

Yoshikawa M, Hirai S, Aizawa A, Kuroiwa Y, Goto F, Sofue I, Toyokura Y, Tamamura H, and Iwasaki Y. A dose-response study with dihydroergotoxine mesylate [Hydergine] in cerebrovascular disturbances. *Journal of the American Geriatrics Society* 31: 1-7, 1983.

More: Dr. Lamb is apologizing for the status quo. In the same column with the Hydergine comment is a question about shingles and acute chronic pain. All he talks about are how long the pain typically lasts — no treatments, nor any comments on the reader's use of codeine and Xanax. He doesn't mention vitamin B_{12}, cyclic AMP, Zovirax nor BHT.

Many professionals and organizations will not tell you about treatments which haven't had the stamp of the American medical establishment. Appreciate the physicians who will. For more information on B_{12}, cyclic AMP and BHT, in herpes and shingles, contact CERI (415-321-CERI). **SWF**

Question: *I have a drug book that says no alcohol-containing over-the-counter medications should be used while taking Hydergine (ergoloid mesylates). My doctor said he didn't think there was any problem with alcohol and Hydergine. What do you say?*

Answer: I agree with your physician. In fact, *liquid* Hydergine is 28.5% alcohol. Throw your "drug book" away. **WD**

Question: *Would Hydergine be okay to take for someone being treated for Candida? I am currently being treated with Nystatin, Caprinex and Capricin.*

Answer: Yes. There are no known adverse drug interactions with Hydergine. The only known contraindication to taking Hydergine is hypersensitivity to ergot alkaloids. **WD**

Question: *I am taking 150 mg of imipramine. Will Hydergine or piracetam have an adverse effect?*

Answer: No.

Question: *My friend and I decided to test the smart drugs Hydergine and piracetam. In fact, all of the smart drugs are widely available over-the-counter in Bangkok, Thailand for a very reasonable price. Because of the cautions in Smart Drugs & Nutrients regarding the up-to-five-fold increased effect when smart drugs are taken in combinations with each other, I arbitrarily decided to start with a fifth of the average suggested intake (two piracetams and one Hydergine). I had to wait about six weeks before I noticed a positive effect. My ability to formulate sentences and my ability to engage in extended verbal presentations increased considerably. I should note that English is not my mother language. I didn't need to take thinking breaks and my responses to questions or problems was almost immediate. I have never had any side effects from the drugs.*

However, I still have the deep feeling that I am not getting all that I could get from smart drugs. It is difficult to explain why I'm thinking this, but it doesn't appear to be the final edge. I would appreciate any recommendations or advice on how to utilize these invaluable drugs to their full extent. I am also interested in knowing how much cigarette smoking and alcohol does/can influence the effect of smart drugs.

Answer: Despite the gradualness of age-related mental decline, our subconscious minds are capable of recognizing the subjective differences between our past abilities and our current ones. This subconscious recognition may be the source of your "deep feeling" that you are still missing something.

The difficulty with smart drugs is that the specific effects of each drug are sometimes unpredictable on an individual basis. The reason recommended dosages are broad, and combination dosages are not given, is that individual variations in responses to each dose are of primary importance. A two-fold variation in a two-drug combination can result in a four-fold variation in the drug ratios. When using multiple drugs, the situation becomes much more complex.

Our recommendations with multiple-smart-drug use is to reassess all the drugs when a new one is added. These same considerations also apply to all the nutrients and neurotransmitters which influence mental function. The combination of phenylalanine and deprenyl, as an example, is much more effective in the treatment of depression than either substance alone.

Question: *Some of the smart drugs (and certain combinations of smart drugs) have profoundly improved my ability to work for long periods and remember data. Others haven't done anything for me. Is this normal?*

Answer: Yes. Each person's unique biochemistry can significantly alter the way in which specific drugs interact with metabolic systems. Furthermore, drugs which target a "weak link" will have more profound impact than ones that miss it. This is true of all drugs, including such common preparations as aspirin, Tylenol and cold remedies. Some researchers have noted that many smart drugs exhibit the "inverted-U-shaped dose-response curve." This effect has also been dubbed "the Goldilocks effect" (not enough is not enough, too much is too much) and "the reverse effect" (too much causes the opposite effect from just right — from the book of the same name, by Walter Heiby). We've seen research that indicates that too much of a smart drug can indeed *decrease* intelligence. The same reverse effect can occur with many common substances. For example, only you can decide how much (if any) coffee is pleasant and stimulating for you. Likewise, there is no perfect dose of any smart drug (or combination) that is right for you. You will need to experiment (under the guidance of your physician, of course) to determine which smart drugs work for you.

It is important to keep in mind that many smart drugs synergize with each other. This means that adding a second drug can make the first one more powerful than it would normally be.

We suggest starting with the smallest doses of any new substance or combination. Gradually increase your dose until you find the right amount. After adding a new smart drug to your regimen, take the time to re-evaluate the dosage of drugs you are already taking.

Question: *What is the best (optimum) dosage for piracetam when taking it in combination with choline, and with Hydergine? Page 31 of* Smart Drugs & Nutrients *states 200 mg of each, page 48 states it's supplied in 400 mg and 800 mg tablets but the usual dose is 2400-4800 mg.*

Answer: First, the dosages of piracetam and choline discussed on pages 31-33 were for a *rat* study, where the dosages were given in mg/kg. This means that each rat was given 200 mg per kilogram of its body weight. This is much different from a dosage of 200 mg. Second, animal dosages cannot be directly converted to human dosages, due to differences in metabolic rate and drug-metabolizing pathways.

It is difficult to recommend optimal dosages of specific smart drugs for individuals, due to biochemical individuality. That's why *ranges* were listed for drugs in *Smart Drugs & Nutrients*. These ranges were based on the least amount of drug required to obtain a therapeutic effect, and the highest amount that has shown benefit without causing significant side effects. As discussed often throughout the book, when combining smart drugs, dosages should be reduced, and increased gradually until maximum benefit is obtained. **WD**

Question: *I have enjoyed reading your newsletters and I have a question I hope you can answer. Can you tell me what drugs are used in other countries to treat Alzheimer's disease, and which are effective? Also, what drugs being investigated in the U.S. seem the most promising?*

Answer: Most of the smart drugs we discussed in *Smart Drugs & Nutrients*, *Smart Drug News*, and *Smart Drugs II* are being used for Alzheimer's disease in one country or another. Although there is no 'magic bullet' for Alzheimer's disease, the most effective drugs are various combinations of Hydergine, piracetam, deprenyl, acetyl-L-carnitine, and nimodipine (a calcium-channel blocker). These last four have their own sections in this book. Pregnenolone, also in this book, looks promising in preliminary research.

Although tacrine (THA) has helped a small percentage of Alzheimer's sufferers, and has recently been approved for use in Alzheimer's disease by the FDA, I think that its significant toxicity should be considered before using it in Alzheimer's disease. It should *never* be used by a normal person as a "smart drug." Another very effective therapy for Alzheimer's disease is *chelation therapy*, a treatment available from members of the American College of Advancement in Medicine (714-583-7666). **WD**

Question: *Have any studies investigated the effects of nootropics (such as piracetam) with brain machines (such as the Alpha-Stim)?*

Answer: Not that I know of. However, studies *have* been done which combined cognition-enhancing substances and memory training [Deberdt, 1992]. In the first study [Israel, *et al.*, 1987; Israel, 1990], the effects of *Ginkgo biloba* extract (GBE) in doses of 160 mg per day, in conjunction with weekly memory training sessions (each of which lasted approximately one hour) were evaluated. There were eighty non-demented subjects in the study, with a mean age of 68 years. Half of each group (placebo and GBE) received memory training. The results of the combined treatments were *additive*.

In a related study on piracetam and memory training, Israel and her colleagues tested varying doses of piracetam (2.4 and 4.8 grams/day) in combination with memory training on 162 non-demented elderly subjects. During the first six weeks, half of each treatment group received memory training. The other half got the training only in the last six weeks. In this study, the effects were again found to be additive. Learning through repetition was improved by the memory training sessions, while piracetam (especially at the higher dose of 4.8 grams/day), consolidated the results of memory training on learning, and improved free recall.

Since the brain machines you mention may have effects similar to memory training, these studies appear to indirectly support the possibility that the combination of smart drugs and brain machines may exhibit synergistic effects. **WD**

Debert W. Interaction between cognitive and pharmacological treatment in age-related cognitive impairments. In: *Treatment of Age-Related Cognitive Dysfunction: Pharmacological and Clinical Evaluation*, Karger, Basel, p. 130-136, 1992.

Israel L. Memory training programs combined with drug therapy in primary care, including patients with age-associated memory impairment. In: *Symposium Piracetam Athens*, by Giurgea CE (Ed.), Madrid, Fundacion Ciencia y Medicina, 22: 17- 22, 1990.

Israel L, Dell'Accio E, Martin G and Hugonot R. Extrait de gingko biloba et exercises d'entrainement de la memoire. Evaluation comparative chez des personnes agees ambulatoires. *Psychol Med* 19: 1431-1439, 1987.

Question: *I don't know which smart drugs will work best for me. I want to take tests as suggested in Smart Drugs & Nutrients by Ward Dean, M.D., and John Morgenthaler. Where can I get such tests? I plan to start with nutrients that I can get without a prescription. I created a computer program that I intend to use for testing for changes in short-term memory. I have taken the test several times a day for over two weeks without taking any smart drugs or nutrients. My scores improved daily during the first week, then they did not change much after that. I think I was learning how to be more effective taking the test during the first week. I average my scores using a four-day moving average so I can graph a smooth XY plot of my progress. My computer test may be an adequate indicator to see improvement, but I'm not sure. There must be tests created by experts, but I don't know where to find them.*

Answer: There are several tests which have been specifically designed to assess the effects of cognitive drugs on AAMI. These are: a French "Batterie de fluidite pour personnes agees," designed by Dr. L. Israel [1988]; a U.S. computerized battery designed by Drs. G. Larrabee and Thomas Crook [1988]; and an Italian battery designed by Dr. G. Savorani and associates [1992]. For information on Dr. Crook's test battery, contact Memory Assessment Clinics, Inc., 8311 Wisconsin

Avenue, Bethesda, MD 20814. We will be describing all of those batteries in future issues of *Smart Drug News*. **WD**

Israel L. Batterie de fluidite pour personnes agees, Paris, *Editions du Centre de Psychologie Appliquee*, 1988.

Larrabee GJ and Crook TH. A computerized everyday memory battery for assessing treatment effects. *Psychopharmacology Bulletin* 24: 695-697, 1988.

Savorani G, Giaquinto S, Cucinotta D, Chiroli S and Salsi A. Computerized cognitive test for evaluating elderly people with mental deterioration. In: *Biomarkers of Aging: Expression and Regulation*, by Licastro F and Caldarera CM, Cooperativea Libraria Universiaria Editrice Bologna, Bologna 40126, Via Marsala 24, Italy, 1992.

More: Most interactive tests and games can be used to track mental performance. As you found, the initial learning curve causes substantial improvement until a performance plateau is reached. After that point, it becomes a statistically meaningful test of certain mental abilities. There may not be that much difference between tests used by scientists, ones you've made up, or such commonly available tests like Tetris, an IQ test, or a plain ordinary typing test. All of these work to some degree to test various combinations of mental abilities. Scientists prefer tests which have been exhaustively analyzed to establish the test's statistical validity within test populations.

Whatever tests you are using for yourself, any repeatable change beyond the learning period is probably significant. The question is, might you be missing something? Is there some mental ability which you are not testing for which might be adversely influenced by a smart drug or lifestyle change?

This issue is best handled by using several tests. Choose one which is obviously spatial, another which is verbal, and another which tests memory abilities. All should be inter- active and have time/performance measures.

One last word of advice: choose tests that you will use regularly. If a test is "too much trouble" to be used regularly, you won't get good data regardless of the quality of the test. **SWF**

Question: *After responding to the ad for deprenyl in the February* Longevity, *I received the following letter from Kerwin Whitnah with ordering instructions for liquid deprenyl from Discovery Experimental & Development company. The price* *seems quite high. Do you know whether the liquid form is more potent?*

Answer: DE&D claims that their version is more efficiently absorbed than the deprenyl that is available in the U.S. by prescription (Eldepryl). The liquid form costs 25¢/mg compared to 20¢/mg for Jumex tablets. However, the liquid form is easier to adjust for more precise doses (1 mg per drop).

Question: *I've started taking deprenyl. Is it necessary for me to stop taking DL-phenylalanine?*

Answer: No, but you might find that you can lower your dose of phenylalanine.

Question: *I've been taking adrenal steroids for asthma on and off for many years Hydergine seems to be helping my asthma. The problem now is how to make getting off the steroids tolerable. I am currently on 15 mg of Triamcinolone. I reduce this dosage by 1 mg per week. I feel exhausted and spaced out a lot of the time. Are there any smart drugs or nutrients that might help? Vasopressin is somewhat useful at my worst.*

Answer: You have a difficult problem. It would certainly be best if you were able to discontinue your adrenal steroids. However, if you have been taking them for many years, it is important to follow the rate that your physician has established for tapering your dose. Have you ever tried Intal (chromolyn sodium) for your asthma? It will not affect the rate of steroid taper, but may eliminate exacerbations of your asthma that would require you to occasionally increase your steroid dose. Use the "spinhaler" rather than the metered dose spray. Another aid to reducing your steroid dependence may be adrenal cortical extract shots. This is a water-soluble extract of bovine adrenal cortex, given intravenously in conjunction with several vitamins and minerals that may restore adrenal functioning and reduce the requirement for high-dose exogenous adrenal steroids (which you are now taking). Call the American College of Advancement in Medicine for the name of a physician in your area who may be able to administer these shots.

Intal (chromolyn sodium) is a drug used to prevent asthma. It may also be obtained by prescription from your physician. **WD**

Question: *What amino acids, foods or vitamins should I not take while using Eldepryl?*

Answer: Eldepryl (deprenyl) is extremely safe and there are no known adverse effects that would be due to any combination of vitamins, amino acids, or other drugs (with the possible exception of simultaneous use of other monoamine oxidase inhibitors).

Question: *In your March, 1992 issue you mention Jumex tablets and Intal. Where would one obtain these? Do you have a source to recommend?*

Answer: Jumex is a brand name for deprenyl, as is Eldepryl. Eldepryl can be obtained by prescription from your physician. Alternatively, liquid deprenyl that appears to be even more pure can be obtained from Discovery Experimental and Development company in Mexico. Their phone number and ordering instructions are listed in the Sources section. Liquid deprenyl is quite stable at room temperature. However, it can be frozen, giving it an almost unlimited shelf life.

Question: *I want to take Hydergine and Eldepryl at the same time. How many milligrams of each would be the right amount day by day?*

Answer: The dosage of Eldepryl (deprenyl) for otherwise healthy adults should be titrated by age (see the dosage schedule below).

Hydergine should be started at low dosage (1-2 mg per day), and increased gradually, to a maximum of about 12 mg per day. I have found, however, that most healthy adults do well on doses of 2-4 mg of Hydergine daily, and do not require the higher doses that may be beneficial in dementing illnesses. **WD**

Recommended Deprenyl Dosages

Age	Dosage	Age	Dosage
30-35	1 mg twice a week	60-65	5 mg every day
35-40	1 mg every other day	65-70	6 mg every day
40-45	1 mg every day	70-75	8 mg every day
45-50	2 mg every day	75-80	9 mg every day
50-55	3 mg every day	80+	10 mg every day
55-60	4 mg every day		

Note: These recommendations are approximate. Individual variation can be substantial.

Question: *Have any studies investigated whether the life-extending effects of chronic food deprivation and deprenyl in mice are synergistic?*

Answer: Not that I know of.   WD

Question: *Can you tell me whether deprenyl and GH3 (Gerovital) taken together would cause the "cheese reaction"? I have not found any studies of the combination of the two, but thought maybe they might cognitively synergize with each other.*

Answer: The "cheese reaction" is a hypertensive crisis that results from a combination of irreversible monoamine oxidase (MAO) inhibitors (many antidepressants are in this class) and simultaneous ingestion of tyramine-containing cheese or red wine. Gerovital will not cause the cheese reaction since it is a *reversible* MAO inhibitor. Deprenyl is an irreversible MAO inhibitor, but is very selective for type-B MAO (MAO-B) and will not generally cause the cheese reaction. In an investigation of deprenyl's use in schizophrenia, very high doses (60 mg/day) were reported to cause partial MAO-A inhibition. Prassad and associates [1988] have reported that patients taking 30 mg/day of deprenyl should be placed on a tyramine-free diet. Since only patients with Parkinson's disease would conceivably be on such a whopping dose of deprenyl (even Parkinson's patients rarely take more than 10 mg/day), healthy people on recommended doses of deprenyl should not be concerned about the cheese reaction.   **WD**

Prassad A, Glover V, Goodwin BL, Sandler M, Signy M, and Smith SE. Enhanced pressor sensitivity to oral tyramine challenge following high-dose selegiline treatment. *Psychopharmacology 95(4): 540-543, 1988.*

Question: *Would there be a problem with taking either tyrosine or DLPA with deprenyl, in the dosages recommended in issues 1 and 6? Also, will deprenyl interact adversely with propranolol (Inderal), antihistamines, or other over-the-counter medications?*

Answer: There are no known contraindications to combining tyrosine or DLPA (DL-phenylalanine) with deprenyl, nor are there any known adverse cross-reactions between deprenyl and the drugs you mentioned.   **WD**

Question: *Sometimes you talk about L-deprenyl and other times you talk about deprenyl. Are they the same drug?*

Answer: Yes. Technically, the drug is called L-deprenyl or (–)deprenyl, because only the left handed isomer (L-form) has the desired biological activity. After mentioning L-deprenyl several times, we feel it is unnecessary, redundant and long-winded to keep saying L-deprenyl, so we merely say deprenyl with the understanding that we are still referring to L-deprenyl. The bottom line: L-deprenyl and deprenyl do refer to the same drug. When isomers do make a difference, we will *always* use the isomer prefix.   **SWF**

Question: *When you become aware of potential suppliers of smart drugs, would you consider testing their service by ordering from them before recommending them? Also, would it be possible for CERI to do lab tests on the products to verify that the drugs are not counterfeit?*

I raise these issues because the deprenyl I ordered from Discovery Experimental and Development company (which I learned of through your newsletter) was not packaged in a box, did not have an expiration date, did not have a lot number stamped on the label, and did not look like any legitimate pharmaceutical I have ever seen. It could easily have been a counterfeit product.

Also, you listed Pharmaceuticals International in your last issue. Although I have successfully ordered from them in the past, they have now proven to be disreputable and I will no longer be doing business with them.

Answer: We appreciate your many concerns. We would like to be able to do the market surveys and chemical assays as you suggest, but we cannot afford to do so under present circumstances. Buying products is expensive enough, but testing pharmaceuticals is a technically difficult and expensive process, especially when chemical standards are not readily available.

Even under ideal circumstances, such a program might easily fail to identify counterfeit products. In the old days, counterfeit products tended to be visually inferior to legitimate products. That is no longer the case. Some counterfeit products are now just as slick and as apparently legitimate as the real thing.

Even professional drug brokers and pharmacists are being fooled by counterfeit products. For optimum effectiveness, we'd need to test continuously, at a cost of hundreds of thousands of dollars.

Discovery Experimental doesn't put their batch numbers or expiration date on the bottles for economic reasons. We were assured, however, that they maintain such records and could pinpoint the batch based on the date of sale of the product. The expiration date depends on environmental conditions: at room temperature, they state that the product undergoes negligible deterioration over 18 months. When refrigerated, it should be several times more stable. Discovery's deprenyl can be frozen, giving it almost unlimited shelf-life. We suspect that figures for longer term stability do not yet exist.

Before we list new suppliers, we require a phone or FAX number and the name of the operations manager, so we can pursue resolution of complaints. Since listing Pharmaceuticals International, we have had a couple of negative reports along with more positive ones. We'd like to hear about the specifics of your problem with them.

Question: *I've been using deprenyl (1-1¼ mg/day) for 1½ years. The Eldepryl from England and the liquid deprenyl from Discovery Experimental in Mexico both give my tongue a definite sensation/taste, but the Jumex I got from International Products in Germany did not. I will enclose a couple of the Jumex tablets if you have any way of determining if they are real deprenyl. The packaging and labeling on the Jumex seemed less professional than the Eldepryl.*

Answer: Please send us the samples. We now have the capability to test deprenyl samples and would like the opportunity. We need 10 tablets or 20 drops *minimum.*

Comment: *Thanks for your answer in the last newsletter. I've enclosed three 5 mg Eldex (deprenyl) tablets for analysis. They were purchased from International Products of West Germany. I believe they may be counterfeit because they taste different from all of my other sources of deprenyl.*

Because Quotaz S.A. might be related to International Products, I haven't yet ordered any of their deprenyl even though their price (10¢/mg) is much less than other sources (20¢- 25¢/mg). Even lower prices may be possible. I have read a couple of reports of deprenyl being purchased in Hungary and Austria for as little as 1-2¢/mg, but was unable to locate the specific source. Pearson and Shaw said that deprenyl is as cheap as 2¢/mg in Italy.

Response: We've sent them off for analysis. However, the tablets were badly crushed in transit and may not be analyzable.

These price discrepancies need to be verified by analysis. If the product is not deprenyl at all, or if it is a racemic mixture of (–)deprenyl and (+)deprenyl isomers, then it's probably not worth the cheap price. If any readers run across any suspiciously cheap deprenyl, please forward us a sample for analysis. **SWF**

Question: *Can I take propranolol (for stage fright) at the same time as low-dose deprenyl? If used infrequently, would this be a problem? My drug book cautions against using them together.*

Answer: There is no reason not to take propranolol and deprenyl together. As long as you are not overdosing on either drug, it will not be a problem. Throw your drug book away.

WD

Question: *Is there any advantage to taking Deaner instead of DMAE from the health food store?*

Answer: Not pharmacologically. Both provide DMAE, which is used for the production of acetylcholine in the brain. The only difference is the acid attached to the DMAE. As a pharmaceutical, Deaner may be subject to higher manufacturing standards than DMAE products found in health food stores. It would depend on the brand and company making it.

Question: *Sheldon Saul Hendler, in his* Doctors's Encyclopedia of Vitamins and Minerals, *says that DMAE should be avoided because of its having lessened lifespan in animal studies. I don't have the citation in front of me as I write, but wondered if you could comment on this.*

Answer: I have not read Dr. Hendler's *Doctor's Encyclopedia of Vitamins and Minerals.* However, in his earlier book, *The Complete Guide to Anti-Aging Nutrients* [1985], he made the same undocumented claim. The only studies that I have seen regarding the effects of DMAE on lifespan are two studies by Hochschild [1973a and 1973b] which showed significant benefits on lifespan and life expectancy (see following figures). One study resulted in a 26% increase in maximum lifespan, with a 39% increase in mean and maximum survival time. The other study resulted in increases of 49% and 11% for mean and maximum survival time, respectively. A significant factor in this study is that DMAE administration was not started until mice were 21 months of age — well past the normal mean lifespan of mice (16 months).

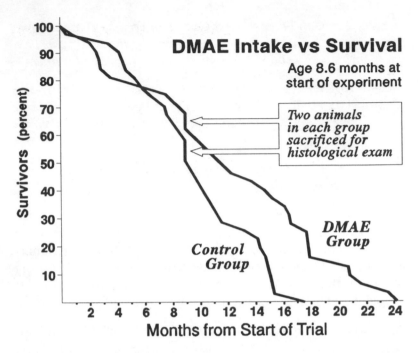

Dr. Hendler is a bright guy, but is extremely conservative when it comes to making recommendations for life-extending supplements. In view of the generally positive effects of DMAE on mental performance in both humans and animals, demonstrated increase of lifespan in animals, overwhelming lack of side effects, and Dr. Hendler's failure to cite the alleged adverse study, I would not be overly concerned about his reservations. **WD**

Hendler SS. *The Complete Guide to Anti-Aging Nutrients*, Simon & Schuster, New York, 78, 251-2, 1985.

Hochschild R. Effect of dimethylaminoethanol p- chlorophenoxyacetate on the life-span of male Swiss Webster albino mice. *Experimental Gerontology* 8: 177-183, 1973a.

Hochschild R. Effect of dimethylaminoethanol on the lifespan of senile male A/J mice. *Experimental Gerontology* 8: 185-191, 1973b.

Question: *Is there anything I should know about taking (or not taking) DMAE in combination with other cognitive enhancers — e.g., Hydergine, PCA (pyroglutamate), piracetam, lecithin (for choline), and Ginkgo biloba?*

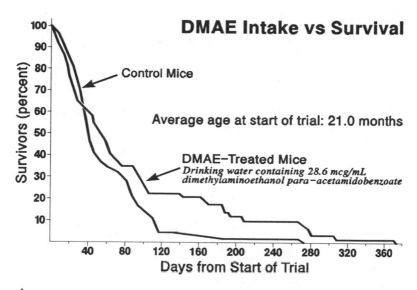

DMAE Intake vs Survival

Control Mice

Average age at start of trial: 21.0 months

DMAE-Treated Mice
Drinking water containing 28.6 mcg/mL dimethylaminoethanol para–acetamidobenzoate

Survivors (percent)

Days from Start of Trial

Answer: Not that we know of, other than our usual cautions of "start low and go slow" when combining various cognition-enhancing substances. Although smart drugs and nutrients as a class are among the safest substances known, we must always be alert for potential adverse effects due to your biochemical individuality, and the known amnestic (forgetfulness-inducing) effect of taking too much of one or more of these substances. See our discussion of "The use of Cerebroactive Drugs" on pages 29-36 of Smart Drugs & Nutrients.   **WD**

More: DMAE (dimethylaminoethanol) is a precursor to choline (trimethylaminoethanol). DMAE and lecithin (phosphatidylcholine) are able to cross the blood-brain barrier to deliver choline to brain neurons. Choline, which is positively charged, is selectively rejected by the blood-brain barrier. The choline content of these two nutrients should be approximately additive.

All of the other substances you mention operate by different mechanisms. Due to the highly interrelated nature of brain functions, however, these substances may act synergistically. Do not underestimate the confounding influences of biochemical individuality in assessing the relative contributions of each of these substances to your program. **SWF**

Question: *I've noticed that recommended dosages for some drugs vary widely from source to source. As an example, I compared the dosages recommended by* Smart Drugs & Nutrients *with those recommended by one of the overseas suppliers.*

Can you comment on these differences? My opinion, based on my personal experience with centrophenoxine, is that a dosage of 3000 mg per day is very high. I have never exceeded 750 mg and even that level caused difficulty in getting to sleep.

Answer: I agree that going much above 1000 mg per day of centrophenoxine is a whopping dose. The recommended dosage range for these drugs should probably be somewhere between the lowest and highest figures. Numerous factors can cause very significant differences in how individuals respond to smart drugs. Age, for example, can strongly influence the amount of drug required. Biochemical individuality is also responsible for large differences.

We used published dose-response studies to set our recommended doses. The overseas company may have used the dose recommendations from specific pharmaceutical companies which are established on a country-by-country basis. Dosages determined by studies of senile or elderly subjects may not be applicable for young, healthy people.

In terms of practical suggestions for our readers, we recommend starting with the lowest recommended dosage. Then increase the dose gradually to find the optimum therapeutic effect. Remember, the optimum dose for you may be much less than the upper end of the recommended dose range. Periodically, and especially when adding new drugs, reinvestigate your ideal dose.

Question: *In your April, 1992 issue, your answer to a question mentioned that the average dose of DMAE might range from 25 mg for a 25-year-old person to 125 mg for a 70-year-old person. I started taking a DMAE-Ginkgo formula from Life Extension*

International which contains 100 mg DMAE bitartrate (with 60 mg of Ginkgo biloba). The recommended dose is two a day. I'm a 33-year-old healthy male who is taking this for life extension and cognitive enhancement. Is this dosage out of line with what might be reasonable, effective and safe? The formula also contains pantothenic acid (80 mg), inositol (25 mg), B₁, B₂, and niacinamide (each 10 mg).

Answer: First, 200 mg of DMAE bitartrate (two 100 mg capsules) is only 37% DMAE. The other 63% is tartaric acid. This means that each capsule contains 37 mg of DMAE for a total of 74 mg in the two capsules you are taking. This is indeed between the 25 and 125 mg mentioned.

Second, the 25 and 125 mg are approximate or average dosages used for purposes of illustration. Some people will experience excessive stimulation from that dose and will judge them too high. Others will take several times those amounts and think them just right. The biochemical individuality that each person brings to their own experience is especially significant in the case of smart drugs. Start with low doses and observe carefully.

One additional warning: the amount of drug in *Ginkgo biloba* herb is highly variable and therefore questionable. There are no formalized standards by which it is measured. In other words, weak herb and potent herb are both measured in total milligrams, but the amount of drug they carry is widely different. When a company says their formula contains 60 mg of *Ginkgo biloba* herb, you have no assurances of how much active drug the product contains. The best Ginkgo products are standardized by potency as well as milligrams. Look for some indication of potency on the label before you buy.   SWF

Question: *I have registered my displeasure with the FDA over the new policy of seizing smart drug shipments from Europe. I'm not sure, however, what to do in the meantime. I have only a few days supply left of piracetam. My Hydergine will run out in a month or so. Are you aware of any alternatives or ways around the current ban?*

Answer: Yes. Hydergine can be obtained by prescription in the United States. If you take the time to find a knowledgeable and sympathetic physician, they could not only prescribe Hydergine but also assist you in the process of importing piracetam for personal use. [See Appendix A for smart drug sources.]

Question: *My check to one of the overseas suppliers was returned with a form letter enclosed telling me that they have been placed on a vaguely defined "FDA Advisory." They suggest that I check with my physician and "check the regulations" again. They even supply an FDA phone number for this purpose. Can you explain what is happening here? Are they looking for some accompanying letter or authorization from a physician?*

Answer: FDA plans and requirements are known only by FDA top brass, and seem to change on their whim. Our recommendations, to arrange overseas purchases in exact accordance with FDA personal-import regulations, are based on taking the FDA at their word. If the FDA is lying to us, then our recommendations will have to change.

Each of the overseas companies are making their own policies in response to the FDA's actions. Interlab is shipping only to people who supply a physician letter or prescription, or to people who will take full financial responsibility for losses due to governmental detentions and seizures. It is up to each person to decide how to proceed: 1) to take the FDA's word that the personal importation regulations are in fact still operating and follow our recommendations, 2) to assume that they are lying and request that shipments be sent without an accurate import declaration, at the customer's risk, or 3) to give up on trying to obtain overseas drugs through the mail.

We have found, however, that if you are following established FDA policies and regulation, and are not violating the law, the FDA will usually cave in if you stand up to them aggressively and assert your rights. As Davy Crockett said, "Be sure you're right, then go ahead."

Question: *You mentioned that the products of six companies are now on import alert. Besides the two you mentioned, which other companies are listed on the ban?*

I've bought products from foreign suppliers and never had problems until recently. International Products returned my last check with the enclosed letter.

I know that smart drugs are available over-the-counter in Mexico. What about Canada? I live close to the Canadian border.

Answer: In addition to InHome Health Services and Interlab, the FDA listed Interpharm, Inc. (Nassau, Bahamas), Northam Medication Service International Pharmacy (Nassau, Bahamas), International Products (Hanover, Germany), Azteca Trio Internacional, S.A. de C.V. (Zona Rio Tijuana, Mexico). CERI lists addresses of such companies only after we have established phone contact with the principals. With international mail-order sales, we insist on being able to talk directly with the person(s) operating the business should any problems arise.

Question: *My order from InHome (vasopressin and Lucidril) was detained by the FDA for sampling of documentation. Their letter claimed that the items were "in violation of 801(a)(3) for a new drug within the meaning of Section 201(p) and not in English per CFR 201.15(c)." Their notice of hearing gives me an opportunity to introduce testimony relating to the admissibility of my order.*

Would it be possible to get an English package insert for the product, and would this bring the product into compliance and allow shipment of the vasopressin? Clearly, the Lucidril will not be allowed in.

Is there anything I can do other than request the FDA to return the shipment and hope to get my money back? The vasopressin is many times cheaper there ($11/5ml vs. $50/8ml for U.S. Diapid).

I would appreciate any advice you could give in this matter. It may be useful to publish this experience in your newsletter, although keep my name and the detention information confidential (I don't want the FDA on my back any more than they are now).

Answer: English package inserts are available or could be made available. Ask for them when you place orders in the future.

Ordering drugs from overseas to save money over U.S. prices is not what the FDA had in mind when they drafted the personal importation regulations. The last thing the FDA wants is for Americans to learn how they are being ripped off by the U.S. pharmaceutical companies. In many cases, the higher prices are a direct result of FDA requirements in this country. Your shipment might get through — if they don't open it, if you give them a real urgent medical reason for needing it, or if they have some reason for not wanting any possible adverse publicity — but it does not fall within their normal discretion.

In actuality, all foreign drugs, whether FDA approved or unapproved, fall under the FDA's legal definition of "new drugs" in section 801(a)(3). Even drugs that the FDA allows to be delivered under the personal importation policy violate that section. The personal import policy merely allows local FDA bureaucrats to not enforce the regulation when it suits them, and details the criteria to be taken into account for specific cases.

Our recommendation: talk to the FDA people directly in charge of making the decision on your shipment. Appeal to their compassion with stories of what the drug has done for you and how you "won't know what to do" if you don't get it. In other words, it's okay to be desperate and scared. Go ahead and get emotional. The last thing a rationally-oriented bureaucrat wants to handle is an emotionally charged situation. Anger may be appropriate to a limited degree, but try to direct it against the "impersonal system that doesn't care about you" rather than the person you're talking to. Make your situation *real*. Also, write your congressperson. Explain to him/her your medical condition, and your requirement for the drug. If you've already used it, tell of your positive experiences. Include a prescription or note from your physician, if possible. Your congressperson will investigate, and will respond to you in writing (Federal officials must respond to Congressional Inquiries promptly). The spineless bureaucrats at the FDA do not want Congressional Inquiries, and will most likely comply with your politely written request.

Question: *I was disturbed to find that the FDA is also targeting vitamins as dangerous drugs that they want to control [Lisa Krieger, Vitamin Peddlers Catch FDA's Eye, San Francisco Examiner, Sunday, May 3, 1992]. At the end of the article there was reference to a "well-organized letter campaign." Do you know anything about this? Who can I get in touch with to participate?*

Answer: The National Labeling and Education Act (NLEA) was passed in 1990. It was an attempt by Congress to encourage and extend the recent trend in health claims on product labels. This trend was encouraged by the National Institutes of Health (*e.g.* the National Cancer Institute and the Federal Trade Commission) and fought by the Food and Drug Administration. The FDA backed down because they recognized that they would lose any legal or publicity battle. Instead, they hunkered down to write draconian regulations for the NLEA. The FDA's NLEA regulations will allow four "health-related claims." All other claims will be illegal. Penalties for making an unapproved claim (even if it is true) will be extremely severe — and there will be *no review of FDA decisions.*

All herbs will be illegal or require a physician's prescription. Vitamins above RDA levels will be illegal or require prescriptions. Some vitamins above RDI levels (proposed levels based on actual consumption instead of what people supposedly need) will be subject to additional regulation. All amino acids will be illegal or require prescriptions. Ethnic foods from South America, Asia and Africa that are not currently listed on the GRAS (generally recognized as safe) list will also be illegal. Foods for which medical claims are made will be illegal or require prescriptions. When your grandmother says, "Eat your fish, Dear, it's brain food," she will be violating FDA regulations and exposing herself and family to FDA enforcement actions. The FDA may not want to go into your house at Thanksgiving to arrest your grandmother, but if Grandma says it on TV and Dad is a fish merchant, watch out!

People to get in touch with:

National Health Alliance (NHA)
P.O. Box 267
Farmingdale, NY 11735
Phone 516-249-7070

Natural Health Care Alliance
3411 Cunnison Lane
Soquel, CA 95073

The obvious place to start is with your representative and senators. There are several ways to proceed. If you don't want to use the phone, write your representative or senator a letter, wait for their inevitable form-letter response, and then send a follow-up letter. This is extremely effective, as it indicates an above-average interest in the issues and usually elicits a personal reply the second time around.

Phone calls add an extra dimension to the influence of a letter. After they have received your letter, call and ask to talk with the legislative aide for health and FDA legislation. This is the person who advises the representatives and senators prior to votes and keeps track of voter sentiments on pending legislation. Express your concerns verbally, ask for information you want, and *thank them for talking to you*. Then send them a letter following up on the conversation.

Such attention to detail, thoughtfulness, and careful follow- up are signs that the legislator's staff pay attention to. For more ways to affect change, see the book *STOP The FDA*, edited by John Morgenthaler and Steven Wm. Fowkes. Single copies can be ordered from CERI at 415-321-2374. **SWF**

Question: *I experience moderate, though chronic, depression. After reading* Smart Drugs & Nutrients, *I ordered some piracetam from one of the overseas suppliers. When I received the* *order, I discovered that I could replace my medication (Xanax) with a low dose (200 mg/day) of piracetam.*

I wanted to discontinue Xanax because I knew it had potential for psychological dependency — although I didn't know how much until I saw the 60 Minutes *segment on Xanax recently.*

After receiving my latest issue of Smart Drug News, *I was very disappointed to learn that the FDA decided to go after the wrong drug. Unfortunately, I only ordered a small quantity of piracetam prior to the FDA import alert.*

Are there any other sources not yet targeted by the FDA?

I am enclosing a SASE for your response. Please respond personally rather than in the next newsletter — I'm concerned that your publications are being monitored by the FDA and any source you publish from now on will be quickly targeted. (The piracetam doesn't appear to help my paranoia.)

Answer: We sympathize with your dilemma. However, things may not be as bad as you think. First of all, the FDA is not as monolithic as you assume. Just because companies have been placed on an import alert doesn't mean that shipments do not get through. Many are getting through. The two most effective strategies are: 1) include a letter within the package that clearly states that the drug is for personal use only, or 2) ship the drug in an unmarked or 'generically' disguised package which lessens the likelihood of attracting the attentions of customs officials. CERI is currently recommending the first option which complies with all laws and regulations regarding access to overseas pharmaceuticals. In your case, your chronic depression could be considered a seriously debilitating illness, for which standard therapy (Xanax) is unsatisfactory. This interpretation of your condition is completely legal, and entitles you to import a personal-use quantity of an overseas pharmaceutical which you believe is a satisfactory treatment. The FDA wants you to have professional supervision for your use of the drug, but they don't always insist especially when the patient appeal is a real tear-jerker. But be prepared to fight and plead for your access, especially in certain backwater ports of entry. Customs inspectors in the Chicago area are notorious for stopping shipments. The FDA personal-importation policy is not a law, it is a regulation, subject to the interpretation and discretion of local FDA administrators. **SWF**

Question: *Is it safe to take piracetam (generic 800 mg or 1200 mg tablets) with an anti-depressant drug like Prozac (fluoxetine 200 mg) which I have been taking daily for 3 months? I also suffer from a degenerative ear disease which renders me profoundly deaf. Is piracetam safe to take without escalating my deafness?*

Answer: There are no known adverse reactions between Prozac and piracetam. In fact, piracetam and may reduce your requirements for Prozac. I have known of several people whose depression was alleviated by piracetam alone, who formerly required Prozac. Piracetam also should not have any adverse effect on your hearing. If anything, it may delay the progression of your condition. **WD**

Question: *What do you suggest I take for depression? Is there anything more potent than Ginkgo/Gotu-Kola, etc.? I would appreciate an answer.*

Answer: If you are clinically depressed, you certainly should be under the care of a knowledgeable physician. There are a number of causes, and a number of potential treatments. As with smart drugs, there is no 'magic bullet,' and the therapeutic approach is often empirical (*i.e.*, 'guesswork'). First, there are the obvious causes: either environmental (*i.e.*, situational), or medical (*e.g.*, hypothyroidism). Often, depression is caused by a neurotransmitter deficiency or imbalance which can be corrected by nutritional or pharmacological manipulation.

For example, if there is a deficit of the stimulatory neuro-transmitter dopamine, this may be corrected by supplementation with amino acids like tyrosine or phenylalanine (up to 2000 mg per day). On the other hand, a mild reversible monoamine oxidase (MAO) inhibitor like Gerovital (see chapter in *Smart Drugs & Nutrients*), or a MAO type-B inhibitor like deprenyl, may help. Improving your sleep patterns using a chrono-regulator like melatonin may improve your sleep and increase your mental and physical energy — common symptoms of depression. Piracetam, deprenyl, and several other smart drugs discussed in this book may be of help (see preceding letter, and see Depression in the Index). Finally, drug therapy with anti-depressants like Prozac is sometimes required. Again, we *strongly* advise medical supervision of all anti-depressant therapies. **WD**

Question: *I have been distressed to find out that the FDA has no intention of allowing tryptophan back onto the market in this country. Tryptophan was the one thing which seemed to help my wife stop her smoking habit. I used it for helping with anxiety and as a mild sleeping pill. Now, of course, we can't get it legally. What stupidity. Alcohol and tobacco kill in a week far more than the adulterated tryptophan ever affected. The FDA didn't take Tylenol off the market forever when some madman poisoned some capsules. The double standard is evident — tryptophan is produced by Japanese companies and Tylenol is made by an American company.*

Answer: We agree that the FDA's continuing ban on tryptophan is a tragic situation. It is a problem, however, to propose a specific reason for the FDA's double standard. The lack of logical rationale to the FDA's arguments and actions can lead to many possible explanations. The FDA may be interested in removing tryptophan so that newly approved serotonin-active drugs can establish market penetration, which they might find difficult with head-to-head competition from tryptophan. The FDA may be exacting a small amount of revenge for losing a battle over tryptophan in the 1970s. Maybe they are trying to establish a precedent for taking all amino acids off the market. We don't know because the FDA is not telling the truth as to why they are keeping tryptophan off the market. Your guess may be as good as any other. Until some kind of official government investigation is conducted into

FDA malfeasance and possible conspiracy, we may never know.

SWF

Question: *In the March issue of* Smart Drug News, *you suggest that over-stimulation due to phenylalanine might be counteracted with serotoninergic enhancement with tryptophan. Isn't tryptophan unavailable?*

Answer: In the U.S., it is unfortunately not available.

Question: *Is it now safe to take tryptophan, obtained from Europe or other sources?*

Answer: Yes, provided it is not from Showa Denko's bad batches. How you would find that out is a problem. Most manufacturers do not like to admit that they were using Showa Denko tryptophan. Although it is now more than three years after the bad batches were produced and Showa Denko is no longer manufacturing tryptophan, there is an off chance that some may have survived the worldwide ban and recall process.

COOH

NH₂

Tryptophan

NH

HO

N-Acetylserotonin

NH

N

H

O

HIOMT
S-Adenosylmethionine

COOH

NH₂

HO

5-Hydroxytryptophan

NH

Melatonin

NH

N

H

O

N-Acetyltransferase
Acetyl-CoA

LIVER   hydroxylation

HO

Serotonin

NH

NH₂

6-Hydroxymelatonin

HO

NH

N

H

O

conjugation
excretion

Although the FDA met with Showa Denko about the tryptophan contamination problem, the proceedings of the meeting are being kept secret. Exact figures of the total amount of contaminated tryptophan sold and the amount recovered by the recall are not being released.

The FDA may have good political reasons for following a policy of obfuscation. The FDA's reasons for maintaining a total ban on tryptophan are scientifically tenuous at best. In addition, the FDA allowed infants and sick and invalid adults to continue to receive Showa Denko tryptophan in infant formulas and total parenteral nutrition (TPN) products for *nine months* after their total recall of tryptophan. No one yet knows how much illness or death resulted from this blunder.

If you can obtain bulk, unprocessed tryptophan from one of the other Japanese companies manufacturing tryptophan (Tanabe, Mitsui or Ajinomoto), you are virtually assured of a quality product. These companies will not ship directly to U.S. customers because of the FDA's permanent ban, but European and Asian companies should be able to buy Japanese tryptophan and ship it into the U.S. under the FDA's personal import policy (if it isn't openly declared as tryptophan on the Customs Declaration Form). Despite the FDA's official position on tryptophan, huge amounts of tryptophan continue to be sold to U.S. animal ranchers. This tryptophan is being produced by a joint Japanese/French manufacturing facility located in Texas.

SWF

Question: *Are L-dopa's side effects really as bad as I've been reading about?*

Answer: The most common side effects of L-dopa are gastrointestinal in nature, and include nausea, vomiting, and loss of appetite. Other side effects like slight headache (usually with over-dosage) are transient, and disappear with continued use or reduction in dosage. There are a number of serious potential side effects of L-dopa, however, which include choreiform or dystonic movements, cardiac irregularities and/ or palpitations, orthostatic hypotension, slowing of the heart,

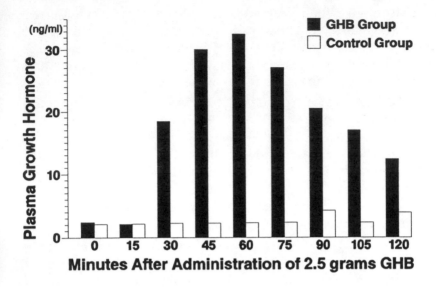

paranoid or psychotic mental changes, ulcers, hemolytic anemia, and agranulocytosis, among others.

With potential side effects like these, L-dopa sounds like a pretty scary drug. However, these side effects were reported in patients with Parkinson's disease, who were taking anywhere from one to eight grams per day! The advanced age of Parkinson patients, combined with the high doses which they take, would naturally cause a greater reported incidence of side effects.

For life-extension and cognitive enhancement purposes, the usual recommended dose is 125-250 mg once or twice daily. These small doses greatly reduce the likelihood of occurrence of any serious adverse effects. I have never noted any such effects in my patients on these low doses. Naturally, L-dopa should be taken under the supervision of a knowledgeable physician who can monitor liver, kidney, cardiovascular and blood-forming functions periodically.   **WD**

Question: *Which is the strongest growth hormone releaser, L-dopa, Eldepryl, or bromocriptine?*

Answer: I am unaware of any growth-hormone-stimulating properties of Eldepryl or Parlodel. Bromocriptine (Parlodel) appears to reduce body fat, cholesterol and triglycerides by inhibiting prolactin [Cincotta and Meire, 1989]. L-dopa is, of course, a powerful growth hormone stimulant [Sonntag, *et al.*, 1982]. Other powerful growth hormone stimulants are niacin (vitamin B3, see figure below) and gamma-hydroxybutyric acid (GHB), a safe hypnotic now outlawed by the Drug Enforcement Administration (DEA) and the FDA   No comparative studies have been conducted on any of these substances, nor have studies been conducted evaluating combinations of these substances.   **WD**

Cincotta AH and Meier AH. Reductions of body fat stores and total plasma cholesterol and triglyceride concentrations in several species by bromocriptine treatment. *Life Sciences* 45: 2247-54, 1989.

Oyama M and Takiguchi M. Effects of gamma hydroxybutyrate and surgery on plasma human growth hormone and insulin levels. *Agressologia* 11(3): 289-98, 1970.

Quabbe HJ, *et al.* Growth hormone, cortisol and glucagon concentration during plasma free fatty acid depression. Different effects of nicotinic acid and an adenosine derivative. *J Clin Endocr Metab* 57: 410-14, 1983.

Sonntag WE, *et al.* L-Dopa restores amplitude of growth hormone pulses in old male rats to that observed in young male rats. *Neuroendocrinology* 34: 163-68, 1982.

Comment: *I am writing in reference to an earlier question in the April 1992 issue of* Smart Drug News, *regarding the comparative growth hormone-releasing effects of various drugs. Dr. Dean said*

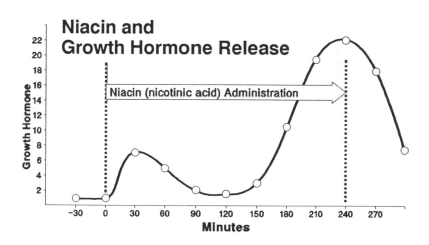

he was not aware of any growth hormone-releasing properties of Parlodel (bromocriptine). Apparently, Parlodel does increase GH levels. In his book, Beyond Anabolic Steroids, *Mauro G. Di Pasquale, M.D., states that, "Some athletes are using Parlodel to increase the endogenous production of both growth hormone and testosterone." He also said, "The reduction in serum prolactin results in an increase in both growth hormone (in those with normal growth hormone levels) and in serum testosterone (secondary to increased levels of luteinizing hormone)."*

Response: Thanks for writing. However, Dr. Hontela tested the effects of Parlodel on growth hormone release in five patients, and found it to have a negligible effect. In four of the patients, the baseline serum growth hormone levels of less than one ng/ml rose to one ng/ml, and in the fifth patient, the baseline level of one ng/ml rose to two ng/ml. Thus, Parlodel does not seem to have any growth hormone stimulating properties. I have seen no other well-documented studies that would counter this finding. Nevertheless, I'm a great fan (and friend) of Dr. Di Pasquale.

For those interested in staying abreast of the latest in athletic-performance-enhancing drugs and nutrients, I strongly recommend his new newsletter, *Drugs in Sports.* Order it from Decker Periodicals, Inc., One James Street South, P.O. Box 620, L.C.D. 1, Hamilton, Ontario L8N 3K7, CANADA. Subscription cost to individuals is $40/year.

Hontela, S, Nair, NPV, Rosenberg, G, Schwartz, G, and Guyda, H. Bromocriptine: Effect on serum prolactin and growth hormone in psychogeriatric howpital patients. *J American Geriatrics Soc*, 1978, 26: 49-52. **WD**

Question: *Can you comment on timing L-dopa supplementation while using smart soft drinks (containing phenylalanine, B_6, fructose, etc.)? I've read that B_6 can cause peripheral decarboxylation of L-dopa, resulting in increased peripheral concentration of dopamine. Is this different than brain dopamine? I'm particularly concerned in the morning, pre-breakfast period, which appears to be the best time to take these supplements (for energy and empty-stomach reasons).*

Biosynthesis of Dopamine, Norepinephrine, and Epinephrine

Answer: This is a very good, but difficult, question. As you can see in the figure, phenylalanine converts to dopamine, which is in turn converted into the excitatory neurotransmitters epinephrine and norepinephrine. The question is — how long does it take for this conversion to occur? The answer is — it depends, both on your individual metabolism, and whether there is anything in your stomach to delay or interfere with absorption. The best way to evaluate your conversion time would be to sequentially measure blood and brain levels of dopamine after a single dose. Obviously, this is impractical (and invasive). The next best way is to take phenylalanine-containing supplements (500-2000 mg) on an empty stomach and time how long it takes for the stimulatory sensation to be perceived (I've heard reports varying from 30 minutes to 4 hours), and how long it lasts. Next, do the same with L-dopa (125-250 mg). Peak levels of L-dopa are usually reached from 30 minutes to two hours after ingestion, and remain for 1-3 hours.

Now you have to decide if you are seeking peak stimulation using both substances (L-dopa *and* phenylalanine), or prolonged stimulation. If you are seeking *peak* stimulation, the ingestion of the two substances should be timed so that peak stimulation occurs at the same time. (Naturally, the doses of both should be reduced to avoid *over*stimulation.) On the other hand, if *prolonged* stimulation is desired, the substances should be taken sequentially, based on the time to onset of stimulation and the duration of the period of heightened awareness. Thus, timing is the key to optimum use of these substances, but optimum timing is not something that can be casually determined.

With regard to the second part of your question, blood and brain dopamine levels are related, but different. We are, of course, most interested in maintaining the *brain* dopamine levels. Vitamin B_6 will cause increased blood dopamine levels, and decreased brain dopamine levels, greatly reducing the effect of supplemented L-dopa. For this reason, many people take Sinemet, which is a combination of L-dopa and carbidopa. Carbidopa enables the L-dopa to more easily cross the blood-brain barrier, and thereby eliminates the concern about the peripheral decarboxylation. **WD**

Question: *I recently heard Dr. Dean and Mr. Fowkes interviewed on KPFA Radio for* Brain Storm *and found the discussion both interesting and informative. Last year I was diagnosed with stage-three breast cancer, which has been treated with the standard 'slash, burn, and poison' method, as well as other more alternative approaches. Much to my distress, I have greatly reduced mental acuity due to chemotherapy. I am also a recovering sugar addict with 25 pounds to lose, and am concerned about my loss of energy and my compromised immune system.*

Can smart drugs be helpful to me? I would greatly appreciate any advice or assistance you could give me.

Answer: Cognitive drugs can partially compensate for reduced mental function from drug toxicity, but the degree of compensation is widely variable from person to person and drug to drug. We can't make specific recommendations, but would like to hear of your results.

Question: *I recently read an article on the drugs Regeneresen and Copolymer 1. I was wondering if you could please send me more information on these two drugs? Do you sell Regeneresen and Copolymer 1, or where can I buy them?*

Answer: Regeneresen is composed of organ-specific ribonucleic acids (RNA) which are injected intramuscularly. RNA are necessary for protein synthesis in our bodies. Unfortunately, RNA concentrations decrease in humans after age 40 [Burger, 1958; Heyden, 1959]. Decreased RNA concentrations, and concomitant decreased protein synthesis, cause decreased efficiency of the entire system, including decreased learning and memory which are closely connected with protein synthesis [Cook, *et al.*, 1963]. Cook and colleagues demonstrated that the learning process in animals is dramatically increased when organ-specific RNA are injected. RNA treatments have been developed for about 80 diseases. These are sold in Germany under the trade name Regeneresen, manufactured by Müller/Göppingen, Cheisch-Pharmazeutische Fabrik, Germany, and may be available from overseas suppliers.

We have no information about Copolymer 1, and would be interested in seeing the article you mention. **WD**

Burger M. Der deoxyribonucleinsaure und ribonucleinsauregehalt des menschlichen gehirns im laufe des lebens. *Z Altersforschung* 12: 133, 1958.

Cook L, *et al.* Ribonucleic acid. Effect on conditioned behavior in rats. *Science* 141: 268, 1963.

Heyden H. Quantitative assay of compounds in isolated, fresh nerve cells and glial cells from control and stimulated animals. *Nature* 184: 433, 1959.

More: Sorry, but CERI does not sell any pharmaceuticals or nutrients whatsoever. Besides being a conflict of interest ethically, product sales would give the FDA legal standing to harass us. **SWF**

Question: *I have written two times to the Pearson and Shaw* Life Extension Newsletter *and did not get a reply. Is the address in* Smart Drugs & Nutrients *okay? P.O. Box 92996, Department*

NF, Los Angeles, CA 90009? Do you have new addresses or phone numbers for them?

Answer: We are in close touch with Durk Pearson and Sandy Shaw. They have assured us that subscribers will receive all issues remaining in their subscriptions. The relocation of their research library has been a monumental task which has disrupted their research and publishing schedule, although they are planning to resume publication in the near future — on an irregular basis. Don't expect a personal reply to any correspondence with them, because they are so busy, but please notify us if any letters sent to them are returned to you. Otherwise, assume that your letters got through. The new address for the *Pearson and Shaw Life Extension Newsletter* is: *DP&SS Newsletter*, P.O. Box 728, Neptune, NJ 07754-0728.

Question: *What information do you have on Trental (pentoxifylline) vs. vinpocetine (Cavinton)?*

Answer: Trental is a prescription drug approved for use in peripheral vascular disease. It acts by increasing the elasticity of red blood cell membranes, allowing them to squeeze through sclerosed blood vessels. In cases of mental impairment due to cerebral atherosclerosis, it is conceivable that Trental could be beneficial by improving blood flow to the brain by the same mechanism. Many people are unable to tolerate Trental because it not infrequently causes significant gastrointestinal side effects.

Cavinton (vinpocetine) is a Hungarian drug not ordinarily available in the United States. As described in *Smart Drugs & Nutrients*, Cavinton acts to improve blood flow by selectively dilating cerebral arteries. It also decreases clotting tendencies of the blood, and enhances oxygen uptake and glucose utilization by the brain. It is relatively devoid of adverse effects, and is effective in doses of 10-15 mg per day.

For those with cerebral circulatory problems, a combination of these drugs would appear to provide greater benefit than either alone. **WD**

Question: *Is there any general (physical and mental) stimulant which is fully as good as caffeine? Many people and books
say that ginseng is as good. But I have not found anything as good
as one Vivarin tablet (caffeine) with 200 mg L-phenylalanine and
one teaspoon of a "high energy" powdered drink. I take these
together, holding them in my mouth so they can dissolve together.
I've read that phenylalanine plays a useful synergistic role in
conjunction with caffeine. My personal experience is consistent
with this observation.*

Answer: Your formula is similar to Pearson and Shaw's Blast
and Fast Blast caffeine-plus-phenylalanine formulas. The
immense commercial success of these formulas certainly attests
to their stimulating effects.

Your "high-energy powdered drink" (if it contains protein) may
be interfering with the efficiency of phenylalanine transport
into the brain. Phenylalanine uses the same enzyme for
transport as other large neutral amino acids (LNAAs), and
competition with other amino acids can seriously reduce the
amount of phenylalanine transported into the brain. For this
reason, phenylalanine should only be used as a smart nutrient
between meals when the stomach is empty of protein.

DLPA (d,l-phenylalanine) is also interesting. It has the
advantage of inhibiting the break-down of naturally produced
brain endorphins and enkephalins (pain killers and euphori-
ants) — and it tastes sweet. DLPA's sweetness makes it easy to
use sublingually. Try a fraction of one capsule under the tongue
when you want a mental lift. DLPA, like phenylalanine, may
also suppress appetite. **SWF**

More: Cylert (pemoline) is a prescription drug that is
indicated for use in attention deficit disorder. Although it is an
amphetamine derivative, it is much safer than most amphetamines and has much less addictive potential (it is a controlled
drug, Schedule IV, by the DEA). The usual dose of 18.75 mg to
75 mg per day gives psychic stimulation for 6-12 hours, often
with a surprising degree of body relaxation. Taken too soon

before retiring, it may cause insomnia. It can promote a higher level of mental concentration in a tired mind. **WD**

Question: *What can I do to relieve insomnia?*

Answer: You didn't say how old you were, how much exercise you get, your state of health, or whether there were any stress factors in your life which may be causing your insomnia. Therefore, this answer will be somewhat general.

First, identify if there are any anxiety-producing situations which may be affecting your sleep and do whatever you can to alleviate them. Second, I recommend some form of rhythmic/aerobic exercise every day. Third, avoid stimulants like caffeine-containing beverages after mid-afternoon.

Finally, you might try taking melatonin. Melatonin is the pineal gland hormone which controls our biological rhythms — especially the wake-sleep cycle. It is very effective in inducing sleep. Melatonin levels decline dramatically with age. Melatonin deficiency is probably the reason older people have difficulty sleeping at night (and remain chronically tired during the day). (See the Melatonin chapter in this book.)

I recommend 3-15 mg of melatonin be taken on an empty stomach about an hour before going to bed.

Another nutrient that may help is gamma-aminobutyric acid (GABA), taken in dosages of about 500-2000 mg about an hour before bedtime. GABA is an inhibitory neurotransmitter which has a calming effect in many people. Herbal sleep-inducing preparations containing valerian and other herbs are available in many health food stores.

Another substance, gamma-hydroxybutyric acid (GHB) (chemically related to GABA) is a great sleep-inducing agent. It increases REM sleep (the most restful sleep), and stimulates the release of growth hormone. It is extremely safe (although it is contraindicated in severe alcoholics, epileptics, or patients with eclampsia, severe hypertension, or bradycardia due to conduction defects). GHB induces a very restful sleep, and reduces body temperature while sleeping (almost a hibernation-like state). Patients also usually awaken sooner than they normally would. GHB seems to be almost an ideal sleep-inducing substance, and may even have life-extension potential, except for one drawback — it's now practically unavailable through legal sources. The FDA and the DEA act as if it is more hazardous than cocaine or heroin. The *Medical Letter*, in a hysterical article which attempted to demonize GHB, concluded that "GHB...has caused severe illness, including seizures and coma. No specific treatment is available, *but all patients so far have recovered spontaneously*" (italics ours).

I do discourage all prescription pharmacological sleep-inducing agents, however, as they contribute to further sleep disturbance.   **WD**

Report: *I have taken 3-6 mg of melatonin (Cardiovascular Research brand, purchased from L&H Vitamins) before bedtime for the past 6 months. A physician friend of mine suggested I try it under my upper lip. I tried one to two mg under my upper lip and had a hard time waking up (some material was still under my lip in the morning), even after taking my usual morning dose of Blast, piracetam, Hydergine and ephedrine. My boss asked me to "wake up" at an 8 a.m. business meeting, and it took several hours to feel awake. The physician suggested using only a small pinch, but that didn't give me the deep sleep that I get with an oral dose. I'm sticking with oral use.*

Answer: Part of the problem may be the solubility of the melatonin. According to Cardiovascular Research, their melatonin capsules are made with free-base melatonin, which is both alkaline and minimally water soluble. Alternatively, melatonin can also exist as an acid-neutralized salt (e.g. melatonin hydrochloride), which should be more water soluble. We haven't seen the research indicating exactly how melatonin is absorbed when taken orally, but it might be absorbed as the free base through the lipid (fatty) phase, or turned into the hydrochloride by stomach acid for aqueous absorption. Because the mouth does not produce acid, sublingual use might necessitate

faster-dissolving melatonin hydrochloride. Free-base
melatonin may cause a "hangover" effect by diffusing too slowly
into the central nervous system through mouth membranes.
(See the Melatonin chapter in this book.)   **SWF**

Question: *What low-risk nutritional supplements or drugs
promote calmness without sedating or impairing mental
function?*

Answer: Anxiety is a diagnosis that is being made with
increasing frequency in the high-stress environment that many
people find themselves in today. One preparation that has
helped a large number of my patients is *adrenal cortical extract*
(ACE). ACE is a water-soluble extract of bovine adrenal cortex
that is extremely helpful in cases of stress or anxiety. In severe
cases, it may be administered intravenously (in combination
with B vitamins and other nutritional substances). Most
physician-members of the American College of Advancement
in Medicine (714-583-7666) are aware of this treatment and will
administer it if required. ACE is also available in a sublingual
form.

Another, more standard, therapy is a medication named Buspar
(buspirone). Buspar is approved by the FDA for the treatment
of anxiety, in usual doses of 10-30 mg per day. It causes *no
sedation*, no euphoria, is not habit forming, and does not
cross-react adversely with other drugs. It usually takes two to
three weeks to take effect, however, so it is not especially
helpful for acute anxiety. Most of my patients who have tried it
report that it makes them feel "normal."   **WD**

Question: *How will Hydergine, piracetam and other smart
drugs mix with anti-inflammatory medications, premarin and
thyroid? I am 68 years old and my memory and alertness are
failing rapidly.*

Answer: Most smart drugs — especially the ones that you
mention — will have no adverse drug interactions with the
medications you are taking. However, if your memory and

alertness are failing *rapidly*, it is possible that you have an as-yet-undiagnosed illness that may be causing these changes.

Too often, older people experiencing rapid mental changes are written off by their family, friends and physicians as "just getting older" when, in fact, a treatable illness is causing these changes. Hypothyroidism is one of the most common causes of memory impairment. See the section on thyroid hormone in *Smart Drugs & Nutrients*. You may need to adjust your dose of thyroid.

WD

Question: *What thyroid replacement does Dr. Dean suggest for low thyroid function? In Broda Barnes' 1976 book* Hypothyroidism *and in Stephen Langer's 1984 book* Solved: The Riddle of Illness, *they both suggest Armour (a combination of T_3 and T_4), but in the dozen papers I've read about subclinical and overt hypothyroidism, they all suggest using only levothyroxine (T_4). They have said most T_3 is converted from T_4 in peripheral/non-thyroid tissue and even with severe hypothyroidism, serum T_3 is often/usually within normal ranges. One paper said they thought it was best not to short-circuit the T_4-to-T_3 conversion (by taking desiccated thyroid with T_4 and T_3) and only T_4 should be used. Another paper said most desiccated thyroid preparations have too much T_3. The only current use of T_3 I've read about is to enhance tricyclic antidepressants.*

Answer: I preferentially use Armour desiccated thyroid, although I have also used Cytomel and Proloid. I avoid Synthroid, which I have found to be less effective than the above three preparations.

WD

Question: *How does the accuracy of Barnes' temperature test for hypothyroidism compare with the TSH assay (elevated TSH above normal range of 0.5-5.0 µg/dl) as an indication of low thyroid function?*

Answer: Although elevated TSH is currently considered to be diagnostic of hypothyroidism, TSH is often normal in cases of subclinical hypothyroidism (as described by Dr. Broda Barnes). The TRH (thyrotropin releasing hormone) stimulation test, which is even more sensitive than TSH, is also often normal in those with subclinical hypothyroidism. As described in *Smart Drugs & Nutrients*, I have found that the patient's symptoms, combined with low basal body temperature, are the best diagnostic criteria for subclinical hypothyroidism. The best confirmation of this diagnosis is a positive clinical response to thyroid replacement therapy. **WD**

Question: *How is piracetam used to treat alcoholism?*

Answer: I was not aware that piracetam was being used to treat alcoholism. However, it's not a bad idea. One of the many adverse effects of chronic excess alcohol use are changes in the brain that are very similar to those of aging [Scheibel, 1979]. In a recent study with rats which were fed alcohol for 12 months (approximately ⅓ of their lives), piracetam reversed many of these changes [Brandão, *et al.*, 1992]. Thus, recovering alcoholics would probably benefit from piracetam. **WD**

Brandão F, Cadete-Leite A, Paula-Barbosa MM. In: *Treatment of Age-Related Cognitive Disorders: Phamacological and Clinical Evaluation*, by Racagni G and Mendlewicz J (eds), Karger, Basel, p. 63-68, 1992.

Scheibel AB. The hippocampus: organization patterns in health and senescence. *Mechanisms of Aging and Development* 9: 89-102, 1979.

Question: *My employers are beginning random urine testing for drugs. I take 1 mg deprenyl (upon waking), 400 mg piracetam (8 a.m. and 5 p.m.), and 1 mg Hydergine (8 a.m. and 5 p.m.). I've read that deprenyl metabolizes into methamphetamine. I have not been under a doctor's care, but I am going to be before drug testing begins. Any words of wisdom to protect myself from hassles? Does piracetam and/or Hydergine cause any problems on drug tests?*

Answer: First some words of wisdom — relax! None of the drugs that you mentioned will be detected with screening tests for illicit drugs. The amount of methamphetamine that theoretically results from deprenyl metabolism is far below the calibration cutoff for these tests, and should not trigger a positive response. Hydergine, which is chemically related to lysergic acid (LSD), is also not detected. The only smart drug

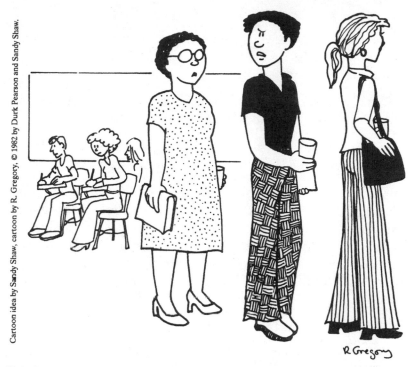

"I don't mind the exam—but I hate these urine tests afterwards, checking for the presence of 'smart drugs'!"

that might rarely cause a response is Dilantin, but only if a very broad screening test is used. However, even Dilantin is seldom detected. I have tested myself several hours after taking all of the above drugs, as well as L-dopa. *None were detected.* However, to be on the safe side — if you are concerned — have your physician enter all of these medications in your health record. Remember — these tests are for detecting illegal drugs. Smart drugs are not illegal. Many common drugs do, however, cause false positives on urine drug screens (i.e., some over-the-counter cold preparations, and ibuprofen, among others). **WD**

Comment: *I'm glad to be getting your newsletter; each issue has had worthwhile information. I look forward to the next one!*

Response: Thanks. We appreciate being appreciated.

Question: *Did Steven Fowkes lay out Dilman's and Dean's new book on a Mac? Looks great. You do great layout. Thanks for the great newsletter.*

Answer: I did the layout for the book, and do it for the newsletter — but on an IBM clone.   **SWF**

Question: *Can you suggest nutrients and chemicals that might help with sustained aerobic exercise in high-altitude conditions?*

Answer: Diamox (acetazolamide), a carbonic anhydrase inhibitor, is indicated for prevention and treatment of mountain sickness. The dosage is 500-1000 mg per day and should be initiated two days before ascending to altitude. Other supplements which may help are vitamin E (400-1200 mg/day), dimethylglycine (50-200 mg/day), and carnitine (500-2000 mg/day).   **WD**

More: Carbonic anhydrase is the enzyme which forces carbonic acid to dissociate into carbon dioxide (CO_2) and water (see illustration). This enzyme allows more carbon dioxide to be exhaled than would otherwise passively dissociate. Inhibition of this enzyme conserves carbon dioxide.

The retention of carbon dioxide causes an increase in acidity and diuresis. Carbonic acid itself lowers pH, and increased excretion of bicarbonate ions tends to cause corresponding loss of sodium and potassium. Loss of these alkaline minerals further exacerbates the possibility of acidosis side effects with acetazolamide.

Acetazolamide is contraindicated in hyperchloremic acidosis, in low Na^+ and/or K^+ states, during kidney or liver dysfunction, and during pregnancy (these folks shouldn't be going on high-altitude mountain climbing expeditions anyway). The drug can cause drowsiness and paresthesia (tingling sensations in the extremities), and its carbonic anhydrase inhibition does not necessarily increase with increasing dose. Because of possible adverse reactions based on personal sensitivity to the drug, it is advisable to start the drug under medical supervision.

Also, see the answer to the following question.   SWF

Question: *I am interested in nutrient and chemical supplements for my upcoming 1993 high-altitude expeditions. Can you suggest supplements that might help with sustained aerobic exercise in the hypoxic conditions found at high altitude?*

Answer: In the chapter on piracetam in this book, we report a study involving young, healthy men, very-low-oxygen conditions, and the protective effects of piracetam. Piracetam has been used for prevention of hypoxia in Himalayan expeditions. Look up "Hypoxia" in *Smart Drugs & Nutrients* for more information on other drugs which are good for hypoxia. Most of these will help alleviate the mental symptoms of low-oxygen conditions.

More: There may be other factors involved besides hypoxia. Background radiation is higher than usual due to diminished density and thickness of the atmosphere between you and the cosmic rays and solar radiation. Increased antioxidant protection may be helpful. Also, with diminished air pressure comes altered oxygen utilization and abnormal gas exchange. The affinity of oxygen and carbon dioxide for hemoglobin is not only concentration-dependent, it is pH-dependent. We were never evolutionarily adapted for survival at 30,000 feet. Metabolic balance between catabolic (acid-forming) and anabolic (alkaline- forming) foods and nutrients may be critical. The pH stress from a metabolic imbalance may adversely influence the pH of the bloodstream and gas exchange.

Unfortunately, blood pH and/or redox tests are too invasive and high-tech for such an environment. However, since blood pH is well-defended by the kidneys, urine pH is probably an accurate indicator of the direction of metabolic stress. If you track your urine pH during the ascent, you can observe not only the degree of acidification from the exertion of the climb, but the degree of compensatory alkalinization during rest and sleep. If your pH becomes chronically acid, you can eat fewer acid foods, and eat more alkaline foods, and take more alkalinizing nutrients. If your pH becomes chronically alkaline, you can do the opposite.

Jan Johnson, who has researched this area extensively, relates a story in which an amateur women's crew team took alkalinizing supplements to counteract the acid stress of long-term rowing (out to Catalina Island and back) to augment their stamina and dramatically improve their racing time. This technique may apply equally well to high-altitude exercise, and maybe to high-altitude rest as well. If you work on this approach, please relate your observations to us. Also, see the answer to the previous question. **SWF**

Question: *I found your acidification/alkalinization article very interesting ("Circadian Metabolism and Consciousness" Smart Drug News, issue #3). I am concerned that my 2-3 times daily usage of smart soft-drinks (choline-type, phenylalanine-type, ephedra-type; all with fructose, citric/malic acid), making my stomach full and acidic, could conceivably have a negative circadian effect. Any tips on keeping the supplement benefits but without all the acidification? At least for the amino acids, I understand the fructose is absolutely necessary for it to be absorbed.*

Answer: Such use could be disturbing your circadian rhythm, but maybe for different reasons than you think. Acidic fruit juices, especially citrus, are *alkalinizing*. They are tart to the tongue, but when their ingredients are *metabolized*, they produce alkaline waste products. I believe this also applies to fruit acids like citric and malic acids, and to carbohydrate sugars.

I have seen individuals (myself among them) who experience specific circadian disturbance to alkaline foods (like fruits and juices) when taken in the morning, as is specified with the Fit-for-Life diet. Other people, especially those who exercise a lot, thrive on such a diet.

If you have difficulty waking up and getting going in the morning, and if you drag on when you eat fruit but not when you eat fried eggs, meat, hash browns or whole grains for breakfast, then the drinks might be a minor problem if you consume them first thing upon waking. If they are, postponing them to just after breakfast, or between breakfast and lunch, might solve your problem. Alternatively, you might also try combining them with more acidic nutrients, like cysteine, essential fatty acids, vitamin A, and vitamin B_{12}.   SWF

Question: *I read with interest your article on "Circadian Metabolism and Consciousness." I would like to order the* Metabolic Balancing Workbook, *pH paper, and newsletter from MegaHealth, but you only mentioned the telephone number. Please let me know their address so that I can order from Europe.*

Answer: Their address was listed at the top of the same paragraph that had their phone number: MegaHealth Society, P.O. Box 60637, Palo Alto, CA 94306 U.S.A.   SWF

Question: *Are any of the cognitive drugs applicable to AIDS dementia?*

Answer: Although peptide-T was developed as an AIDS drug, it is chemically related to both vasoactive intestinal peptide (VIP) and vasopressin, and has shown an uncanny ability to alleviate a number of AIDS-related neuropsychological symptoms, including dementia. People with AIDS (PWAs) using peptide-T often report dramatic improvement in mental function (*i.e.*, memory, concentration, reasoning, etc.) and improvement in such AIDS-related symptoms as weight loss, diarrhea and fatigue. It is known to pass the blood-brain barrier.

Peptide-T is not easy to come by. Nor is it cheap. At present, peptide-T has yet to be approved in any country and is made by only a handful of pharmaceutical companies. Currently, the only sources for the drug are AIDS Buyers Clubs. The price ranges from $300-$350 for a 50-day supply. The dose currently employed by most underground users is 5 mg via subcutaneous injection (½ cc), but Dr. Candace Pert's original study used intravenous administration. An ongoing study at UCLA is now investigating intranasal (2 mg three times per day) use. There has been a lot of criticism of intranasal administration by underground proponents of peptide-T. However, anecdotal accounts from participants and physicians involved with the study have been quite encouraging.

Beyond peptide-T, numerous cognitive drugs are able to compensate for dementia, but none are known to deal with the underlying causes of AIDS. Presumably, unless one treats AIDS, the problem will continue to become more severe, despite short-term gains from cognitive drug use.

Question: *What about the dangers of vasopressin? I read somewhere that it has caused heart attacks but no mention was made (in an anti-smart-drug article) about whether this was with prolonged usage or with occasional usage. I'm assuming that no one should use it frequently unless they need it for a medical condition besides memory loss.*

Answer: Vasopressin causes temporary constriction of small blood vessels (arterioles) and therefore should not be used by anyone with hypertension, angina, or atherosclerosis. It is a very safe medication for anyone else. Since its vaso-constricting effects are transient, prolonged usage will not cause an increased risk of adverse effects in those for whom the drug is *not* contraindicated.   **WD**

Question: *What can you tell me about pregnenolone? All that I know about it appeared in the enclosed article. Do you know where it might be available?*

Answer: See the pregnenolone section in this book and our pregnenolone article in *Smart Drug News* #2 for further information. We do not have any sources yet, but it used to be available 40 years ago and may still be, somewhere in the world. Now that new uses are being discovered and demand is rising, sources will spring up. We'll announce them as we hear of them. See the tearout card at the front of this book for subscription information.

Question: *Your article on steroid precursors (pregnenolone) was quite interesting. I have always heard that taking anabolic steroids causes the body to shut down its natural production resulting in testicular atrophy. Could such a feedback mechanism also operate with DHEA or pregnenolone? What are the relative risks of taking these compounds?*

Answer: Anabolic, androgenic (male), estrogenic (female), and progestoid (gestational) steroid hormones do cause negative feedback inhibition. Steroid precursors like cholesterol, pregnenolone and DHEA, which do not have much steroid activity, do not. The pituitary gland produces releasing hormones (peptides) which stimulate the testes, ovaries, and adrenal glands to produce steroid hormones. These steroid hormones circulate through the bloodstream to the hypothalamus, in the brain, which then sends a feedback signal to the pituitary, saying "make more" or "make less." So feedback inhibition by steroids is controlled by the hypothalamic sensitivity to the steroid in question. Fortunately, the hypothalamus is quite specific. It does not recognize cholesterol, pregnenolone or DHEA as steroids and so does not down-regulate the pituitary's releasing hormones when these steroid precursors increase. Therefore DHEA and pregnenolone have few, if any, adverse side effects.   **SWF & WD**

Question: *I'm taking 600 mg DHEA daily under my doctor's supervision. What's the best blood test to measure DHEA, free DHEA or DHEA sulfate? Do symptoms associated with DHEA include sweats and extreme sleepiness?*

Answer: Both DHEA and DHEA-sulfate (DHEA-S) decline significantly with age [Carlstrom, *et al.*, 1988]. Professor Carlstrom [1989] advised me that "DHEA-S is the most significant marker for clinical evaluations (it is far more stable than DHEA, which has considerable diurnal variations)." However, he also believes that in some cases, the ratio between the two is of value, since the balance between the unconjugated (DHEA) and conjugated (DHEA-S) is affected by thyroid and hepatic factors.

I have just finished reading the definitive book on DHEA—*The Biologic Role of Dehydroepiandrosterone (DHEA)* by Mohammed Kalimi and William Regelson. It is published by Walter de Gruyter, Inc., Hawthorne, NY, 1990, and costs $242.90! No DHEA-related symptoms as you are having are described in the book.   **WD**

Carlstrom K, Brody S, Lunell NO, *et al.*. Dehydroepiandrosterone sulphate and dehydroepiandrosterone in serum: differences related to age and sex. *Maturitas* 10: 297-306, 1988.
Carlstrom K. *personal communication*, 1989.

Question: *I recently heard that the DEA plans to put DHEA on the controlled list as an androgenic steroid. Can you explain what this means, and what is the difference between androgenic and anabolic?*

Answer: We spoke with a DEA spokesperson who denied that there were any plans to classify DHEA as a scheduled (controlled) steroid. Although DHEA does have weak androgenic activity, it is not sufficient to be medically classified as an androgenic steroid. The DEA, however, may be lying to us about their real intentions, and may indeed classify it as a dangerous steroid despite the lack of medical or scientific grounds.

Androgenic refers to a testoid or masculinizing influence; anabolic refers to the process of cellular building or rebuilding (whereby nutrients are assimilated into body structure). **SWF**

More: At a recent scientific conference, I spoke to a researcher from the Veterans Administration who has done a great deal of basic research on the cognition-enhancing properties of DHEA. He said that it is now extremely difficult to obtain DHEA, even for legitimate researchers. The reason, he believes, is that the DEA contends that DHEA can be used in the manufacture of anabolic steroids and this has dramatically restricted its availability. **WD**

More: The DEA considers possession of illegal-drug precursors to be a crime comparable to possession of the illegal drug itself. **SWF**

Question: *Thank you for the informative newsletter,* Smart Drug News. *It is great! I appreciate any and all information that I can obtain on the treatment of Alzheimer's. I recently purchased a copy of the book* Reducing the Risk of Alzheimer's *by Dr. Michael A. Weiner, written in 1987. My inquiry to the publisher (Stein and Day, Scarborough House, Briarcliff Manor, NY 10510) about more recent material was returned to me with no forwarding address. Can you tell me if Dr. Weiner has written further, or how to get in touch with Stein and Day?*

Answer: Yes, Dr. Weiner is still actively researching and writing. He has another book, *Weiner's Herbal,* which discusses the chemistry, pharmacology, and uses of over 200 herbs. Many of these herbs have cognition-enhancing effects, as well as many other beneficial and therapeutic effects. His other book, *Reducing the Risks of Alzheimer's Disease* is also still available, and includes a chapter on the benefits of chelation therapy. These books can be obtained from Quantum Books, 6 Knoll Lane, Suite D, Mill Valley, CA 94941, 415-388-1006, FAX: 415-388-2257. Dr. Weiner is involved in another interesting project, which we'll announce as soon as we can. **WD**

Correspondence

Please send your questions to: CERI Q&A, P.O. Box 4029, Menlo Park, CA 94026-4029, U.S.A. You may also FAX them to CERI Q&A at 415-323-3864, or phone them to us at 415-321-CERI. Questions are answered in future issues of *Smart Drug News*.

Part IV:

Appendices

Part IV: Appendices

Product Sources

In early printings of *Smart Drugs & Nutrients* we listed several overseas mail-order sources for smart drugs. Since then, the situation surrounding the availability of smart drugs has changed dramatically. The FDA issued import alerts on a half-dozen overseas suppliers, and the original sources we listed have either gone out of business or changed their addresses. The FDA's policy toward smart drugs also seems to be in a state of flux. We are also discovering new sources on an ongoing basis. Due to these unpredictable and unstable conditions, we decided not to list any overseas mail-order sources here, as they are likely to change after printing. We do, however, list a number of U.S. sources for smart nutrients.

To obtain a current listing of overseas sources (ten as of the date of publishing of this book), send the tearout card at the front of this book to CERI and request the product sources list. Include $2 for postage and handling (the list is free to *Smart Drug News* subscribers). CERI's list is updated on a monthly basis (subscribers automatically receive all updates), so you can get the latest information on overseas smart-drug sources.

Cognition Enhancement Research Institute
P.O. Box 4029-2014, Menlo Park, CA 94026-4029 U.S.A.
Phone: (415) 321-CERI FAX: (415) 323-3864.

We also strongly encourage you to subscribe to CERI's newsletter, *Smart Drug News*. The U.S.A. price is $44 per year for 10 issues ($46 Canada/Mexico, $55 overseas). Or, you can phone or FAX CERI for credit card purchases.

Smart Drug News covers the latest smart drug and nutrient research. In the Q&A section, subscribers can get their questions answered by experts on smart drugs.

Smart drugs are available in many foreign countries. Pharmacies in Mexico, for example, often stock most of the drugs listed in this book. U.S. Customs has traditionally allowed personal importation of foreign drugs for personal use. Some people have told us that they combine their vacation plans with buying trips. Other countries where readers have reported purchasing smart drugs include: Thailand, Italy, Spain, and Belgium.

In this appendix, we include a few of the most reliable sources for smart nutrients in the United States. These sources cannot sell drugs which either require a prescription in the U.S. (like Hydergine), or are not available in the U.S. (like piracetam).

Smart Nutrients by Mail

Klaire Laboratories
13 West Seminole, San Marcos, CA 92069
Phone: (800) 533-7255 or (619) 744-9680

Klaire Laboratories (also known as Vital Life or Prime Life) sells a line of supplements (including magnesium glycinate) especially designed for allergic or chemically-sensitive individuals. Their products contain no sugars, starches, soy, fish oil, acacia, wheat, corn, milk, yeast, artificial sweeteners, artificial coloring, or salicylates. They produce top quality, scientifically formulated, non-reactive and price competitive supplements.

Life Services Supplements, Inc.
3535 Highway 66, Building #2 , Neptune, NJ 07753
Phone: (800) 542-3230 or (908) 872-8700
(use (800) 345-9105 in Canada)

Life Services is a mail order company and worldwide licensee to market and manufacture all 28 Durk Pearson and Sandy Shaw Designer Food™ formulations. All ingredients are purchased from high-quality sources. Life Services guarantees same-day shipping on all orders received prior to 4 p.m. east coast time. They also will conduct searches for you of computer databases such as Medline, the database of the National Library of Medicine, and Embase, the European medical database.

NutriGuard Research
P.O. Box 865-A, Encinitas, CA 92023
Phone: (800) 433-2402 or (619) 942-3223

NutriGuard sells a comprehensive line of high-quality nutritional supplements that includes vitamins, minerals, amino acids, and essential fatty acids. The products are available in capsules, tablets, and powders. NutriGuard generally has low prices. They have the lowest price we have seen for 50% phosphatidyl choline. Technical data sheets are available which describe the thinking behind the formulations.

Smart Products
870 Market Street, Suite 1262-SD, San Francisco, CA 94102
Phone: (800) 858-6520 or (415) 989-2500

Smart Products offers most of the nutrients listed in this book and in *Smart Drugs & Nutrients* including acetyl-L-carnitine, arginine pyroglutamate, and DMAE. They have great prices, fast service, a free newsletter, books, videos, and the complete line of Pearson & Shaw products. They also offer an entire line of cognition-enhancing formulations. Even if you don't order from Smart Products, we suggest you get on their mailing list for their newsletter.

Smart Buys at Health & Vitamin Stores

Health-food and vitamin stores offer a wide variety of smart nutrients. Many stores offer high-quality products from these two nutrient manufacturers.

Source Naturals
P.O. Box 2118, Santa Cruz, CA 95063
Phone: (408) 438-6851

Source Naturals manufactures the Mental Edge™ formula, one of the first brain formulas available. Many people report that Mental Edge and Source's new MegaMind™ both have very noticeable cognitive effects. These formulas include many of the smart nutrients covered in *Smart Drugs & Nutrients* and this book: acetyl-L-carnitine (ALC), N-acetyl-L-tyrosine, L-pyroglutamic acid, DMAE, and ginkgo biloba 24% extract.

We often stress that a substance that works well for one person may do nothing at all for someone else. Each individual must try a few different smart nutrients to find what works. The broad spectrum of nutrients in MegaMind and Mental Edge increases the likelihood that the consumer will experience a cognitive effect, yet the formulas offer the convenience of a single tablet. For the "do-it-yourselfer", each of these nutrients is also available from Source Naturals as individual supplements.

Source Naturals' line of brain nutrition products is continuously being expanded. The formulas are available in health food and vitamin stores throughout the country, and/or can be ordered by a store for you.

All the tablets are vegetarian, made with highest quality ingredients, and the lowest possible amounts of excipients and binders. Source's tabletter is an artist, and the tablets dissolve in your digestive tract, not in the bottle.

TwinLab
Ronkonkoma, NY 11779
Phone: (516) 467 3140

TwinLab is the manufacturer of a complete line of nutritional products in capsules. Their products are available in most health food and vitamin stores. Their quality is uniformly excellent.

More Drug & Nutrient Sources

Healing Alternatives Foundation
1748 Market Street, Suite 204, San Francisco, CA 94102
Phone: (415) 626-2316

HAF carries an extensive selection of vitamins and nutrients which would be of interest to those utilizing a natural approach to cognitive enhancement.

Carl Vogel Foundation
1413 K Street NW, 14th Floor, Washington, DC 20005-3405
Phone: (202) 289-4898

This club stocks a number of nutrients and vitamins.

LifeLink
445 Lierly Lane, Arroyo Grande, CA 93420
Phone: (805) 473-1389

LifeLink provides promising therapies for AIDS which include concentrated hypericin extracts and soluble melanins.

PWA Health Group
31 W. 26th Street, 4th Floor, New York, NY 10010
Phone: (212) 532-0363

PWA Health Group is a not-for-profit organization formed to supply people with AIDS with hard-to-get AIDS treatments. They carry some of the smart drugs and nutrients covered in this book.

Information Sources

Smart Drug News

Smart Drug News is published ten times annually by the Cognitive Enhancement Research Institute (CERI). Edited by Steven Wm. Fowkes, with Medical Editor Ward Dean, M.D., and Contributing Editor John Morgenthaler, *Smart Drug News* is devoted exclusively to covering the latest research on smart drugs and cognitive enhancement. The "Question & Answer" column allows subscribers to get their real-life questions answered by Fowkes, Dean, and Morgenthaler. Write to CERI, P.O. Box 4029, Menlo Park, CA 94026-4029, or call (415) 321-CERI (321-2374). Credit-card orders can be phoned in or FAXed to (415) 323-3864. One-year (10 issue) subscription are $44 ($46 Canada/Mexico, $55 overseas) and include CERI's product sources list and directory of physicians. Please also refer to the tearout card at the front of this book.

Smart Drugs & Nutrients

Smart Drugs & Nutrients: How To Improve Your Memory And Increase Your Intelligence Using The Latest Discoveries in Neuroscience, by Ward Dean, M.D., and John Morgenthaler, published by Health Freedom Publications, Menlo Park, CA (see last page of this book to order).

"...a bible for the smart drugs set."

— Los Angeles Times Magazine

"An excellent introduction to the field of cognition-enhancing compounds... Well-written and easily understood, even by people who do not have specific training in medicine."

— Giacomo Spignoli, M.D., Ph.D.
Pharmacology Research Director,
L. Manetti–H. Roberts & Co.

"A dirty little book."
— Dan Rowland, Compliance Officer, Los Angeles District
Office, Food and Drug Administration

The Age Reduction System

The Age Reduction System, Dr. Richard C. Kaufman, Ph.D.,
1986, published by Rawson Associates, New York, NY. This
very-well-researched book covers much basic information
about life extension.

A Remarkable Medicine Has Been Overlooked

A Remarkable Medicine Has Been Overlooked, by Jack Dreyfus,
1981, published by Simon and Schuster, New York, NY. This
painstakingly researched book is the fruit of Dreyfus' 20-year
effort to alert the medical profession and the world at large
about the benefits of phenytoin (Dilantin). The book has a
great 2140-reference bibliography and review that covers some
of the most important discoveries about this incredible drug.

Biological Aging Measurement

Biological Aging Measurement: Clinical Applications, by Ward
Dean, M.D., 1988, published by The Center for Bio-Gerontology, P.O. Box 11097, Pensacola, FL 32524. This book was
written for biomedical gerontologists and life extension
experimenters to evaluate the efficacy of experimental
life-extension/age-retarding programs by measuring
age-related biomarkers. It describes over 200 physiological,
biochemical and psychometric parameters that change with age
(see order form on the last page).

*"A valuable reference...the first time that anyone has seriously
proposed the use of these systems to measure the aging processes."*
— Johan Bjorksten, Ph.D.

*"Highly recommended for anyone involved in anti-aging therapy
or experimentation."*
— Roy Walford, M.D.

"The most pertinent life-extension book available."

— John A. Mann

Brain Boosters

Brain Boosters, by Beverly Potter, Ph.D., and Sebastian Orfali. Preface by Ward Dean, M.D., 1993, published by Ronin Publishing, Berkeley, CA. A pioneering look at the substances that have a positive effect on the performance of the human brain. Describes the most important pharmaceutical, vitamins, nutrients and herbs used to boost brain power. Includes a directory of life-extension doctors and clinics.

The Complete Guide to Anti-Aging Nutrients

The Complete Guide to Anti-Aging Nutrients, by Sheldon Saul Hendler, M.D., published by Simon and Schuster, 1985. This is a very comprehensive, even-handed evaluation of nearly every nutrient purported to have anti-aging effects. It is encyclopedic in scope and provides a wealth of scientific references.

Dialog

Dialog Information Services, 3460 Hillview Ave., Palo Alto, CA 94304. Phone: (415) 858-2700. Dialog is the world's largest online information service. This means that people use their computers to call Dialog and search hundreds of databases for answers to their questions. Dialog is expensive and takes some time to learn to use, but it offers a sister service called *Knowledge Index* that is much easier to search and is available at a reduced cost. Much of the research we did to write this book was done by conducting more than a hundred searches of *MedLine* (the on-line version of the National Library of Medicine) and *Embase* (the European on-line medical library) with *Knowledge Index*.

If you have been diagnosed as having a disease and want to know about the latest treatments or want to know about research on a particular drug, you can have a search of MedLine (or any other online database) done by a reference librarian at many libraries. There are also companies which will conduct an online search for you for a fee, including Life Services at (800) 542-3230.

Drugs Available Abroad

Drugs Available Abroad, by Jerry L. Schlesser (Ed.) and Derwent Publications, Ltd., 1991, published by Gale Research Inc., Detroit, Michigan. Covers over one thousand drugs that are approved in other countries but not approved in the United States. Contains hard-to-find therapeutic information, drug actions, precautions, dosages, etc.

Forefront

Forefront — Health Investigations, edited by Steven Wm. Fowkes. This newsletter reviews medical technologies rarely covered anywhere else. While oriented towards life extension, the journal goes far afield to cover the work of the likes of Emanuel Revici (the New York physician responsible for a whole theory of biology based on the body's acid and alkaline balance), alternative cancer treatments, chelation therapy, AIDS therapies, and political issues. The writing is excellent and easy to understand. Six-issue subscription $18 by third class mail, $21 by first class mail, $21 in Canada, $25 by overseas airmail, from MegaHealth, P.O. Box 60637, Palo Alto, CA 94306, Phone: (415) 949-0919.

How to Live Longer and Feel Better

How to Live Longer and Feel Better, by Linus Pauling, 1986, published by W. H. Freeman, New York, NY. Pauling is the two-time Nobel Prize-winning biochemist reviled by the medical establishment for his research into the health benefits of vitamin C and other antioxidants. But according to Pauling's peers,that is, nutritionally-oriented physicians and scientists,he is a gifted scientific pioneer. Crick and Watson credit Pauling with the co-discovery of the structure of DNA. Pauling would probably have shared Crick and Watson's Nobel Prize had he been able to join them in their research. However, he was denied travel visas during the McCarthy era due to his pacifist beliefs and political activities. A reporter researching Pauling for *Penthouse* magazine in the late 80s talked to many of the top physicists and biochemists in the U.S. They all agreed that Pauling is one of the greatest minds our country has produced.

How to Live Longer and Feel Better outlines Pauling's personal life-extension program and includes easy-to-understand explanations of the mechanisms of aging and the actions of vitamins, 30 pages of scientific references, and the eye-opening story of the "controversy" about vitamins.

Life Extension

Life Extension: A Practical Scientific Approach, by Durk Pearson and Sandy Shaw, 1982, published by Warner Books, New York, NY (see back page to order). Pearson and Shaw made the term "life extension" a household word with their best-seller, their many television appearances, and their incredible recall of scientific research. This 858-page book addresses all aspects of aging, including sexuality, depression, cancer, heart attack risk reduction, and intelligence increase. Written in a friendly and sometimes humorous style, *Life Extension* has practical 'how-to' suggestions for slowing down the rate of aging in your own body — all based on documented scientific research. The book is fun to read and also makes a great reference manual. It's designed to be used by both professional people and non-professionals. *Life Extension* has an excellent index, and many health problems or questions are listed with several pages to which you can refer.

Pearson and Shaw delayed publication of *Life Extension* for a year because Warner Books thought that the 96 pages of scientific references were unnecessary. Warner Books ultimately relented to avoid the lawsuit that the authors initiated to ensure the inclusion of their bibliography. Obviously, the science behind their work is important to Sandy and Durk. Ten years after *Life Extension* was published, the ideas that "free radicals cause aging" and "vitamins fight disease" have become mainstream. *Time* magazine and ABC's *Nightline* have run major stories. Yet Durk and Sandy are rarely credited as the harbingers of this revolution.

Mind Food and Smart Pills

Mind Food and Smart Pills, by Ross Pelton, R.Ph., Ph.D., with Taffy Clark Pelton, 1989, published by Doubleday, New York, NY 10103. This book presents a compendium of vitamins, herbs, and drugs that can work wonders for the human mind. From antioxidants like vitamin C and selenium which counteract the damaging effects of free radicals, to herbs like ginseng and Ginkgo biloba that can combat brain aging, each supplement is covered in detail. It is a predecessor to *Smart Drugs and Nutrients*, and has a great deal of valuable information not covered in other books.

The Neuroendocrine Theory of Aging

The Neuroendocrine Theory of Aging and Degenerative Disease, by Vladimir M. Dilman, M.D., Ph.D., D.M.Sc., and Ward Dean, M.D., published by the Center for Bio-Gerontology, P.O. Box 11097, Pensacola, FL 32524. (See back page to order). Professor Dilman is one of the most widely known scientists in Russia and the republics of the former Soviet Union. Dilman theorizes that aging is a disease process that everyone who reaches maturity suffers from, and that most age-related disease conditions are merely manifestations of this one underlying 'super-disease.' This concise and highly technical book proposes unique therapeutic regimens to slow and even reverse aging, and to treat age-related diseases.

Orphan Drugs

Orphan Drugs, by Kenneth Anderson and Lois Anderson, 1987, published by The Body Press, Los Angeles, CA 90048. *Orphan Drugs* is like a *Physicians' Desk Reference* for over 1500 drugs that are available outside the U.S., but which, for various reasons, have not been 'adopted' by U.S. pharmaceutical companies. The Andersons include two separate indexes —

one for the various trade and chemical names under which the drugs are sold, and one for the symptoms and diseases that the drugs are used to treat. There is a great directory of drug manufacturers, and the book also has an excellent description of how the FDA works (and doesn't work) in this country.

Physicians' Desk Reference

Physicians' Desk Reference, annual, published by Medical Economics Company, Oradell, NJ. The *PDR* is a guide for physicians to the use of drugs that the Food and Drug Administration approves for use in the U.S. Only FDA-approved drug uses are listed here, and this book is the sole source of information about pharmaceuticals for many physicians. You can find the *PDR* in most libraries. Each drug's listing includes contraindications, dosage information, drug interactions, and adverse effects.

Smart Life Special Interest Group

NSS Smart Life Special Interest Group, P.O. Box 620123, Woodside, CA 94062, (415) 851-4751, FAX: (415) 851-1265. This special interest group is sponsored by NSS, Inc. As far as we know, this is the only special interest group on smart drugs and life extension that is open to the public. The group has monthly meetings with presentations on a wide variety of topics. NSS sponsors an annual conference related to sexuality, life extension and performance enhancement held in the San Francisco Bay area. If you would like to attend (or start an interest group in your area) please contact Kathryn Roberts at NSS Seminars, Inc.

Smart Nutrients

Smart Nutrients, by Abram Hoffer, Ph.D., and Morton Walker, D.P.M., 1993, published by Avery Publishing. This ground-breaking book reveals the more complex nutritional demands of the brain: vitamins B_3 and C, along with zinc, chromium and many other vitamins and minerals that are important in the prevention and treatment of disabling brain disorders. It outlines a program readers can follow to prevent and correct degenerative brain diseases as well as to improve already strong mental capacities.

STOP the FDA

STOP The FDA: Save Your Health Freedom, with articles by Linus Pauling, Ph.D., Ward Dean, M.D., Senator Orrin Hatch, Durk Pearson & Sandy Shaw, and many others. Edited by John Morgenthaler and Steven Wm. Fowkes, 1992, Health Freedom Publications, Menlo Park, CA (see back page to order). This book is a call to activists to turn the tide from mandatory medical mediocrity brought about by FDA regulation of the medical industry. *STOP The FDA* may anger you, it will definitely inform you, and it will arm you with the information you need to counteract the FDA's war on American health freedom.

Index

FDA and, 229
hyperactivity and, 118
intelligence increase and, 114
life extension effects of, 122
non-verbal intelligence and, 19
prenatal use of, 20-21
violence and, 117-118

W

Walters, Barbara, 2
Wedbush Morgan Securities, 21
Wong, Cliff, 2

Z

Zatosetron, 85
 5-HT$_3$ and, 87
 AAMI, treatment for, 87
 ondansetron and, 87
Zinc, 273
 Alzheimer's disease, and, 133

About the Authors

Ward Dean, M.D., graduated from the U.S. Military Academy, West Point, New York. He served as an infantry officer for six years, during which time he was an instructor at the U.S. Army Ranger School and combat advisor to the Vietnamese Rangers. He received his M.D. degree from Han Yang University, Seoul, Korea. During seven more years of service, Dr. Dean participated in a number of classified missions as Flight Surgeon for the *Delta Force*, America's top-secret counter-terrorist unit.

Dr. Dean is now the Medical Director of the Center for Bio-Gerontology in Pensacola, Florida. He has published more than 70 articles and reviews in professional journals, and is the author of *Biological Aging Measurement — Clinical Applications* [1988], co-author of *The Neuroendocrine Theory of Aging and Degenerative Disease* [Dilman and Dean, 1992], and co-author of *Smart Drugs & Nutrients* [1990].

John Morgenthaler is a science writer and publisher in San Francisco, California. He has degrees in psychology and computer science and has research experience in the field of artificial intelligence. John has also launched several successful business ventures. He has been researching smart drugs and nutrients since 1980.

John is the co-author of *Smart Drugs & Nutrients* [1990] and *Smart Drugs II: The Next Generation* [1993]. He is also co-author (with Steven Wm. Fowkes) of *STOP The FDA: Save Your Health Freedom* [1992]. John has appeared on the *Today Show*, *Larry King Live*, *20/20*, and *Phil Donahue*, and has been interviewed in *Time*, *Playboy*, *Washington Post*, *USA Today*, *New York Times*, *Los Angeles Times*, *San Francisco Chronicle*, *The Economist*, *Rolling Stone*, *Mademoiselle*, and many others.

Steven Wm. Fowkes is Executive Director of the Cognitive Enhancement Research Institute (CERI), and Editor of *Smart Drug News*. His degree is in organic chemistry. Since 1983, he

About the Authors

has been Director of the MegaHealth Society and Editor of their newsletter, *Forefront — Health Investigations*. Steve is author of several books and magazine articles about health issues, and edited Dilman and Dean's *Neuroendocrine Theory of Aging and Degenerative Disease*.

Steve has extensive experience designing supplement formulas, several of which have become multi-million sellers. He has been researching and using nutrient-based cognitive technologies for twenty years.

Order Books by Phone
from CERI

☎ Call (415) 321 CERI

Smart Drugs & Nutrients, by Ward Dean, M.D. and John Morgenthaler, $12.95

Smart Drugs II, by Ward Dean, M.D., Steven Wm. Fowkes, and John Morgenthaler, $14.95

STOP the FDA, articles by Linus Pauling, Ph.D., Ward Dean, M.D., Senator Orrin Hatch, Durk Pearson & Sandy Shaw, and many others. Edited by John Morgenthaler and Steven Wm. Fowkes, $9.95

The Neuroendocrine Theory of Aging and Degenerative Disease, by Vladimir M. Dilman, M.D., Ph.D., D.M.Sc., and Ward Dean, M.D., hardback $65

Biological Aging Measurement: Clinical Applications, by Ward Dean, M.D., $39.95

Life Extension: A Practical Scientific Approach, by Durk Pearson and Sandy Shaw, hardback, $22.50

Wipe Out Herpes with BHT, by John A. Mann and Steven Wm. Fowkes, $4.95

Mind Food and Smart Pills, by Ross Pelton, R.Ph., Ph.D. with Taffy Clark Pelton, $12.95

100% Money Back Guarantee